Caregiver

In

Gastroenterology

The complete Guide

MARTIN STERLING

Table of contents

« Working in gastroenterology is like being a detective of the digestive system: you investigate what's going out, guess what's coming in, and hope it all stays inside! »

Introduction: Why this book?

- The important role of the gastroenterology orderly

The importance of the role of the gastroenterology nursing auxiliary is undeniable, and constitutes one of the pillars of the smooth running of this medical service. As a healthcare professional, the orderly is on the front line of day-to-day patient care, playing a crucial role that goes far beyond simple technical care. In a department as specific as gastroenterology, where the pathologies treated directly affect vital aspects such as digestion, nutrition and elimination, the caregiver becomes a real player in patient comfort and well-being.

The role of the nursing auxiliary begins as soon as patients are welcomed. He or she is often the first person to make direct contact, providing a reassuring first impression to often anxious patients. The caregiver must be able to adapt his or her approach to each individual, whether young adults with inflammatory bowel disease, elderly people with chronic illnesses such as cirrhosis, or patients with digestive cancer. Each pathology implies specific care, and the caregiver must quickly understand the particular needs of each patient to adjust his or her care.

In this context, the caregiver plays a key role in daily management, whether for hygiene, comfort or clinical monitoring. Patients hospitalized in gastroenterology can be confronted with difficult situations: stomas, incontinence, vomiting and recurrent abdominal pain. These symptoms, which are sometimes taboo and resented, require professional but sensitive support. The nursing auxiliary becomes not only a care technician, but also a psychological support, helping patients to regain a form of dignity despite the alterations in their physical state.

In addition to hygiene care, the nursing auxiliary also plays a key role in monitoring clinical signs. By observing patients' progress on a daily basis, they are often the first to detect subtle but significant changes: a change in stool frequency, an unusual appearance of vomiting, or signs of deterioration in general condition. Their close proximity to the patient enables them to quickly spot signs of worsening pathology, and to pass on this information to the nursing team for rapid intervention. This "watchdog" role is essential, because in gastroenterology, critical situations such as digestive haemorrhage or intestinal perforation can occur suddenly.

Gastroenterology nursing assistants are also distinguished by their involvement in technical care, particularly in the preparation and follow-up of endoscopic examinations. Colonoscopies, gastroscopies and other investigations require physical preparation, often stressful for the patient. The nursing auxiliary has the delicate task of preparing patients for these examinations, ensuring their comfort and understanding of the process. They then accompany them during the post-examination period, providing care and comfort in the face of fatigue or possible complications. In this way, they become a key player in the care chain, guaranteeing patient safety and well-being at every stage.

In addition to these technical aspects, the role of the gastroenterology orderly has a profoundly human dimension. They need to be empathetic and good listeners, and sometimes have a great capacity to manage the emotions of patients and their families. Digestive pathologies, often chronic or incapacitating, can significantly alter patients' quality of life, provoking anxiety, frustration and sometimes isolation. The caregiver, through his or her daily presence and proximity, is often the one who offers moral support, a smile or a reassuring word, helping to lighten the burden of the disease.

It's clear, then, that the gastroenterology orderly does more than just perform repetitive tasks. He or she is a key player in the department, capable of combining technical expertise, clinical vigilance and humanity. They help to coordinate care, ensure patient comfort, and play a central role in the smooth running of care. Their impact on patient care is profound, as they ensure continuity of care and support at all times, making hospital stays more bearable for patients faced with pathologies that are often severe and complex.

•   The specifics of gastroenterology: a field rich in diversity
Gastroenterology is a particularly broad and diverse field of
medicine, touching on many essential functions of the human
body, including digestion, nutrient absorption and waste
elimination. This field of medicine is distinguished by the
multiplicity of organs involved - from the esophagus to the
rectum, via the liver, pancreas, stomach and intestines. This
anatomical diversity implies complexity in pathologies,
treatments and care, making gastroenterology a specialty as
technical as it is rewarding. Working in a gastroenterology
department exposes you to a wide range of medical situations,
from benign conditions to disabling chronic illnesses, and even
life-threatening emergencies.

One of the major specificities of gastroenterology is the wide
variety of pathologies it encompasses. Chronic inflammatory
bowel diseases (such as Crohn's disease or ulcerative colitis) are
striking examples. These conditions, often diagnosed in young
patients, require long-term management, involving
immunomodulatory treatments, sometimes complex surgery, as
well as ongoing psychological and nutritional support. Alongside
these pathologies are functional digestive disorders, such as
irritable bowel syndrome, which, although less serious, can have a
major impact on patients' quality of life. These disorders require
careful, personalized management, combining a therapeutic
approach with moral support, as symptoms can be aggravated by
stress and other psychological factors.

The liver, the central organ of metabolism, also plays a major role
in gastroenterology, with a variety of pathologies ranging from
viral hepatitis to alcoholic or metabolic cirrhosis. These liver
diseases, often asymptomatic in their early stages, sometimes
progress to advanced and irreversible stages, with serious
complications such as liver failure or liver cancer. The
management of these diseases requires constant vigilance, with
particular attention to early signs of deterioration, such as the
appearance of ascites or hepatic encephalopathy. What's more, the

treatment of these patients may require specialized interventions, such as ascites punctures or liver transplants, illustrating the technical nature of this specialty.

Cancerous diseases also play an important role in gastroenterology, with cancers affecting the entire digestive tract and associated organs. Cancers of the colon, rectum, stomach, pancreas and liver are among the most common, and require multidisciplinary management combining surgery, chemotherapy, radiotherapy and palliative care in advanced cases. The therapeutic approach in gastroenterology therefore involves close coordination between gastroenterologists, surgeons, oncologists and support care teams. The diversity of surgical treatments, ranging from bowel resections to colectomies, illustrates the extent to which this specialty encompasses varied and often complex procedures, requiring great rigor in pre- and post-operative management.

In addition to serious pathologies, gastroenterology is also concerned with more common but often disabling disorders, such as gastro-oesophageal reflux, gastric ulcers and gallstones. Although these conditions are more common, they are no less delicate to treat, as they closely affect patients' daily quality of life. For example, a patient suffering from severe gastro-oesophageal reflux may be severely hampered in his or her daily activities and eating habits, requiring rigorous therapeutic management combined with appropriate nutritional advice. Similarly, biliary lithiasis may require surgical intervention such as cholecystectomy, a frequent but not risk-free operation.

Another aspect that makes gastroenterology particularly rich is the importance of diagnostic examinations and techniques specific to this specialty. Digestive endoscopy, whether upper (gastroscopy) or lower (colonoscopy), is one of the most common and essential examinations in gastroenterology. It not only allows us to visualize the interior of the digestive tract, but also to take biopsies, remove polyps and treat certain lesions. These examinations, although routine in practice, require meticulous preparation of the patient, often with specific diets or purges, and close monitoring after the procedure to avoid complications. The nursing auxiliary plays a key role in preparing and accompanying patients before, during and after these procedures, ensuring their comfort and safety.

Finally, gastroenterology is distinguished by its holistic approach to the patient. Digestive pathologies are often associated with other co-morbidities, such as diabetes, obesity or cardiovascular disease, which can exacerbate digestive disorders. It is therefore essential to take a holistic approach to patient management, working closely with other medical specialties to ensure comprehensive, coordinated care. For example, an obese patient suffering from gastro-oesophageal reflux disease will benefit not only from drug treatment, but also from dietary advice and possibly surgical management (such as bariatric surgery) to treat the underlying cause of the reflux.

• Objectives of this book: To inspire, train and guide
The aim of this book is threefold: to **inspire**, **train** and **guide** caregivers, whether they are at the start of their career or already experienced, through a realistic and detailed vision of everyday life in a gastroenterology department. By bringing together practical information, experience-based advice and sound medical knowledge, this book aims to become a valuable resource that illuminates every stage of patient care, while offering insights into the personal and professional commitment of caregivers.

Inspire: reveal the vocation and impact of the profession

The first objective is to inspire those considering or already working in gastroenterology, by highlighting not only the technical nature of this profession, but also its profoundly human aspect. Caregivers play an essential role in the care of patients suffering from pathologies that are often incapacitating, sometimes chronic, and that touch on intimate and vital aspects of their lives. Through personal accounts, real-life situations and concrete examples, this book aims to remind us that this profession, though sometimes trying, is also a vocation rich in encounters, challenges overcome, and moments of satisfaction.

Every day spent at the bedside is an opportunity to make a difference, whether it's giving special attention to an anxious patient before an examination, or providing moral support to a patient going through a difficult period. This book shows how the caregiver, through his or her caring presence and daily gestures, makes a fundamental contribution to improving patient well-being and recovery. By recounting positive experiences and illustrating the concrete impact of this profession on patients' lives, the aim is to encourage future orderlies to enter this specialty with passion and determination.

Training: imparting essential knowledge and skills

The second objective is to provide **training** for nursing assistants, by offering them a comprehensive, practical guide covering all aspects of work in gastroenterology. The book is intended to be a veritable toolbox, containing basic medical knowledge, techniques specific to this specialty, and methods for improving the quality of day-to-day care.

Gastroenterology care is often complex, requiring ongoing training to master technical procedures such as ostomy management, nasogastric tube management and post-endoscopy monitoring. The book will detail these procedures, explaining step-by-step what the orderly needs to do to ensure patient safety and comfort. In addition to the technical aspects, training also includes learning how to communicate with patients who may be anxious or suffering from chronic and serious illnesses. Knowing how to listen, soothe and reassure is just as essential a skill as the application of care itself.

By providing a sound theoretical framework and practical examples, this book prepares caregivers to deal with a wide variety of situations, from managing gastrointestinal emergencies to caring for patients at the end of life. Each chapter is designed to provide immediately applicable knowledge, while prompting wider reflection on how to constantly improve care practices.

Guiding: support for day-to-day and long-term challenges

Finally, this book aims to **guide** caregivers, not only in the management of day-to-day care, but also in the development of their career and professional resilience. Working in a gastroenterology department can be demanding, both physically and emotionally, and it's essential that orderlies know how to manage the challenges they face. This book will help them do just that, with strategies for overcoming stress, preventing burn-out and achieving work-life balance.

It's important for nursing assistants to be aware of the evolution of their profession and the possibilities for professional advancement. This book will guide them as they explore the different career prospects open to them, whether to specialize further in certain aspects of gastroenterological care, or to move into training, research or coordinating positions.

What's more, in an ever-changing medical context, this book offers pointers for navigating the new challenges posed by technological advances and changes in care protocols. From the use of new medical devices to the management of increasingly well-informed patients, caregivers must continually adapt their practices. This guide will provide the keys to staying up-to-date and competent, while reinforcing the importance of collaboration with other members of the care team.

In short, this book's mission is to inspire, educate and guide gastroenterology orderlies by providing them with an overview of their profession, while giving them concrete tools to excel in their daily practice. It's a book that celebrates the importance of their role, while preparing them for the many challenges they will encounter in this demanding but rewarding specialty.

Chapter 1

Understanding gastroenterology: general framework and main pathologies

1 The gastroenterology department: a complex and diversified specialty

- Definition and role of gastroenterology in the healthcare system

Gastroenterology is a medical specialty dedicated to the study, diagnosis, prevention and treatment of diseases of the digestive system. This field encompasses a wide range of essential organs, from the esophagus to the anus, as well as accessory organs such as the liver, pancreas and bile ducts. As a specialty, gastroenterology plays a central role in the healthcare system, as it affects functions vital to the human body, including the digestion of food, the absorption of nutrients, and the elimination of waste. Dysfunctions of the digestive system can have a major impact on patients' quality of life and, in the most serious cases, can be life-threatening.

Gastroenterology is essential to the detection and treatment of many diseases, some of which are extremely common, such as gastro-oesophageal reflux disease, gastric ulcers and alcohol-related liver disease. At the other end of the spectrum, this specialty also deals with complex and serious pathologies such as digestive cancers, chronic inflammatory bowel disease (IBD), and liver cirrhosis, which require long-term, sometimes multidisciplinary, care. The diversity of pathologies managed by gastroenterology makes it an indispensable discipline, not only for the prevention of digestive diseases, but also for their treatment and long-term follow-up.

Gastroenterology's role in the healthcare system is not limited to the management of acute or chronic conditions. It also plays a fundamental role in the early detection of serious illnesses, thanks in particular to diagnostic tools such as colonoscopy and gastroscopy. These examinations enable direct visualization of the inside of the digestive tract, identifying abnormalities such as polyps or ulcers, and taking biopsies to confirm a diagnosis of cancer or inflammatory disease. This preventive role is particularly crucial in the case of colorectal cancer, one of the most common and potentially fatal cancers, but which can be effectively treated when detected at an early stage.

The preventive role of gastroenterology also extends to the management of liver disease, which is on the rise, particularly as a result of obesity, diabetes and excessive alcohol consumption. Non-alcoholic steatohepatitis (NASH), for example, has become a major cause of cirrhosis and liver failure. Gastroenterologists are at the forefront of screening and management of these conditions, helping to prevent their progression to more serious complications, such as liver cancer or the need for liver transplantation.

Another essential aspect of gastroenterology's role in the healthcare system is the management of chronic diseases of the digestive tract, such as Crohn's disease and ulcerative colitis. These conditions, which often affect young people, require constant monitoring and adjustment of treatments as symptoms evolve. Gastroenterologists work in close collaboration with other healthcare professionals - nurses, dieticians, psychologists - to ensure comprehensive patient care that goes beyond simple drug treatment. Dietary support, monitoring nutritional deficiencies and psychological support are just some of the dimensions that illustrate the complexity of this specialty.

In addition to diagnosis and treatment, gastroenterology plays a central role in the management of digestive emergencies, which can represent an immediate threat to patients' lives. Digestive haemorrhage, intestinal obstruction or intestinal perforation are critical situations requiring rapid intervention to avoid serious or even fatal complications. The ability to react quickly in these contexts, by performing therapeutic endoscopies to stop bleeding, or by organizing emergency surgical management, makes gastroenterology a discipline where decisions must be taken efficiently and precisely.

From a broader perspective, gastroenterology also contributes to public education and awareness of lifestyle habits that can influence digestive health. An unbalanced diet, a sedentary lifestyle, alcohol consumption and stress are all factors that can lead to digestive disorders. Gastroenterologists therefore play an educational role, advising patients on how to prevent these conditions through lifestyle changes. Increasingly, this specialty is taking a preventive approach, focusing on long-term digestive health rather than simply managing symptoms.

Finally, gastroenterology is also a specialty at the heart of many medical innovations. Technological advances, such as the endoscopic capsule, interventional endoscopy and new biological treatments for chronic inflammatory bowel disease, have transformed the way digestive diseases are diagnosed and treated. This specialty is evolving rapidly, and gastroenterologists must constantly train in new techniques and treatments to offer their patients cutting-edge care. In this way, gastroenterology not only meets patients' current needs, but also anticipates future challenges by integrating medical innovations and adapting to demographic and epidemiological changes.

- Structure and organization of a gastroenterology department

The structure and organization of a gastroenterology department are essential to ensure efficient, coordinated patient care. This medical service is based on a rigorous organization, where the skills of several healthcare professionals are integrated to meet the complex needs of patients suffering from digestive diseases. The gastroenterology service is generally structured around several complementary departments, each with specific roles and functions, ranging from diagnosis and treatment to post-operative follow-up and chronic disease management.

A gastroenterology department generally includes **an** inpatient **unit**, where patients requiring ongoing care are admitted for varying periods of time, depending on the severity of their condition or the complexity of their treatment. In this unit, patients may be hospitalized for a variety of reasons, such as management of acute complications (digestive hemorrhage, occlusions, exacerbations of chronic inflammatory bowel disease), preparation for and recovery from digestive surgery, or monitoring of heavy drug treatments (chemotherapy, biotherapy). The inpatient unit is an intensive care unit where the focus is on continuous monitoring of patients' clinical signs and vital parameters.

At the heart of this unit, the role of the care team is crucial. It is made up of nurses, orderlies, gastroenterologists, dieticians, physiotherapists and, occasionally, psychologists. Each professional has a well-defined mission, but all work closely together to ensure comprehensive patient care. For example, gastroenterologists make diagnoses, establish treatments and perform specific technical procedures, such as endoscopies or ascites punctures. Nurses and orderlies, for their part, monitor patients on a daily basis, administer treatments, ensure their comfort, and provide hygiene and support. The dietician, for his part, plays a decisive role in adapting the patient's diet, taking into account the specific constraints of each digestive pathology.

The gastroenterology department also boasts a specific **technical platform**, where diagnostic and therapeutic examinations are carried out. This includes several endoscopy rooms, where procedures such as colonoscopy and gastroscopy are performed, as well as more specialized explorations such as echo-endoscopy and endoscopic retrograde cholangio-pancreatography (ERCP). These examinations enable us not only to visualize the interior of the digestive tract and associated organs, but also to intervene to remove polyps, dilate stenoses or treat digestive haemorrhage. The technical platform is a highly specialized facility, where coordination between the gastroenterologist, the specialized nurse and the nursing auxiliary is essential to ensure patient safety and comfort, as well as the smooth running of procedures.

In addition to the technical platform, some gastroenterology departments have an **outpatient unit**, where patients come for consultations or treatments that do not require prolonged hospitalization. This unit is particularly important for patients with chronic diseases, such as Crohn's disease or ulcerative colitis, who require regular monitoring and frequent adjustments to their treatment. Ambulatory care also includes procedures such as setting up infusions for intravenous treatments, or carrying out follow-up biological and radiological examinations. This ambulatory approach allows for more flexible and less restrictive management for patients, while guaranteeing high-quality medical follow-up.

The structure of the gastroenterology department also often includes a **digestive surgery unit**, as many digestive pathologies require surgical intervention. This unit works closely with gastroenterologists to manage pathologies such as digestive cancers, intestinal occlusions or complications of chronic inflammatory bowel disease. Digestive surgeons perform tumor resections, stomas, intestinal anastomoses and liver transplants. The link between the medical and surgical gastroenterology teams is essential to ensure continuity of care, from diagnosis to post-operative follow-up.

Another fundamental element of the department's organization is the **multidisciplinary consultation**, where several specialists meet to discuss complex cases. These meetings enable us to adopt a global, concerted approach, integrating the opinions of gastroenterologists, surgeons, oncologists, radiologists, and sometimes psychologists and nutritionists. This collaborative approach is essential in the management of digestive cancers or serious chronic diseases, as it enables personalized treatment plans to be drawn up, tailored to the specific needs of each patient.

Finally, the **educational dimension of** the gastroenterology department is also a key aspect of its organization. Patients suffering from digestive pathologies, especially chronic diseases, often need training in how to manage their disease. The department therefore sets up therapeutic education workshops, where patients learn how to manage their diet, watch out for signs of relapse, or take care of their stoma. These workshops are led by specialized nurses, dieticians and other professionals, and aim to make patients more autonomous in managing their health.

- Collaboration between caregivers, nurses, doctors and other professionals

Collaboration between orderlies, nurses, doctors and other healthcare professionals is central to the smooth running of a gastroenterology department. This cooperation is essential to ensure comprehensive, high-quality care tailored to patients' needs. In gastroenterology, where pathologies are often complex and care varied, the complementary skills of each professional are essential to ensure personalized and effective follow-up. Harmonious teamwork makes it possible to meet the technical and human demands imposed by digestive diseases, while creating a caring and supportive environment for patients.

The nursing auxiliary occupies a unique position in this collaborative dynamic. On the front line of care, they are close to patients. He or she is the one who assists patients in their daily lives, providing hygiene, comfort and assistance with basic needs. Their role is essential, as they are often the first to observe subtle clinical signs that may herald a deterioration in a patient's state of health. Thanks to this close, trusting relationship, the caregiver acts as a "watchdog", passing on his or her observations to nurses and doctors so that rapid, appropriate decisions can be taken. The caregiver's ability to communicate effectively with the nursing team is crucial to ensuring responsive care, particularly in the event of a gastroenterological emergency, such as digestive bleeding or decompensation of a chronic disease.

Nurses, for their part, are key players in the day-to-day management of patients. They administer treatments, perform specific technical care, such as fitting nasogastric tubes or managing stomas, and monitor vital parameters. Their role goes beyond the technical, however, as they are also responsible for coordinating care between the various medical and paramedical teams. Nurses work in close collaboration with orderlies, delegating some care to them while ensuring supervision and regular transmission of medical information. They also act as a link between patients and doctors, explaining treatments, answering patients' questions, and ensuring that medical orders are applied precisely. This direct collaboration with the nursing assistants creates a smooth and harmonious care environment, where everyone knows their role and responsibilities, while contributing to the overall well-being of the patients.

The **gastroenterologist** is often at the center of diagnostic and therapeutic management. He or she is responsible for assessing symptoms, making diagnoses, and defining the treatment plan. Collaboration with other healthcare professionals is essential to ensure continuity of care and an individualized approach. In consultation with nurses and care assistants, the doctor relies on their daily observations to adjust treatments and refine diagnoses. For example, depending on signs reported by the caregiver or nurse, such as a change in bowel movements or recurring abdominal pain, the doctor may decide to order additional tests, such as a colonoscopy or abdominal scan. This communication between doctors and nursing staff is crucial to ensuring rapid response and adapting care to patients' changing needs.

The doctor also works closely with other **specialists**, such as digestive surgeons, oncologists and radiologists. As digestive pathologies often require multidisciplinary approaches, these professionals regularly consult each other to discuss complex cases and develop common therapeutic strategies. In the case of colon cancer, for example, the gastroenterologist, oncologist and surgeon will work together to plan the stages of treatment, integrating chemotherapy, surgery and possibly palliative care. This multidisciplinary collaboration ensures integrated, comprehensive care, with each professional contributing his or her expertise to offer patients the best possible treatment options.

In addition to the interactions between doctors, nurses and orderlies, other healthcare professionals play a central role in a gastroenterology department, such as **dieticians** and **psychologists**. Patients suffering from digestive diseases often need specific nutritional advice, whether to manage an ostomy, follow a residue-free diet before a colonoscopy, or adapt their diet to their pathology. The dietician collaborates with the rest of the team to draw up suitable food plans and monitor patients' nutritional status. The dietician is also involved in educating patients on good long-term dietary practices, a crucial aspect especially for those suffering from chronic diseases such as Crohn's disease or liver cirrhosis.

Psychologists also play an essential role in supporting patients, especially those with serious or chronic illnesses, who may experience anxiety, depression or difficulty coming to terms with their condition. Collaboration with the rest of the team ensures that patients' mental health is monitored as a whole, integrating psychological support with medical treatment. Indeed, many digestive disorders are influenced by stress and emotions, and psychological support can play a decisive role in recovery or long-term disease management.

Finally, collaboration is not limited to direct care. **Communication between the various healthcare professionals is** reinforced by regular meetings, where patients' cases are discussed, therapeutic decisions are taken in concert, and care is adjusted. These multi-disciplinary meetings provide a forum where everyone can share their observations and knowledge, helping to improve patient care and ensure a coherent, comprehensive approach.

2 Overview of the main pathologies treated in gastroenterology

- Inflammatory bowel diseases (Crohn's disease, ulcerative colitis)

Chronic inflammatory bowel diseases (IBD), mainly represented by Crohn's disease and ulcerative colitis (UC), are chronic intestinal disorders characterized by persistent inflammation of the digestive tract. These two diseases share many features in common, but also differ in important ways in terms of localization and clinical presentation. They significantly affect the quality of life of patients, who often have to cope with disabling symptoms, heavy treatment and sometimes surgery. Although the precise causes of these diseases remain poorly understood, they are considered to be autoimmune conditions in which the immune system inappropriately attacks intestinal tissue.

Crohn's disease

Crohn's disease can affect any part of the digestive tract, from the mouth to the anus, although it is most often localized in the terminal ileum (the last portion of the small intestine) and the colon. It is characterized by transmural inflammation, i.e. it affects all layers of the intestinal wall, which explains the diversity of its complications. This inflammation can lead to ulcerations, fistulas)abnormal connections between different parts of the digestive tract, or between the intestine and other organs), and abscesses.

Symptoms of Crohn's disease vary from patient to patient, but often include intense abdominal pain, chronic, sometimes bloody diarrhea, and significant weight loss. Fatigue is another major symptom, accentuated by chronic inflammation and nutritional deficiencies linked to poor nutrient absorption. The course of the disease is marked by periods of inflammatory flare-ups, alternating with phases of remission of varying duration. These flare-ups can be triggered by infections, stress, certain foods, or sometimes for no apparent reason.

Complications of Crohn's disease are numerous and can include intestinal obstructions caused by narrowing of the digestive tract (strictures), fistulas between the intestine and other organs (such as the bladder or skin), or intestinal perforations. These complications often require surgical intervention. Unfortunately, even after surgical resection of part of the intestine, Crohn's disease tends to recur in other areas of the digestive tract, complicating its long-term management.

Hemorrhagic rectocolitis (UC)

Unlike Crohn's disease, ulcerative colitis only affects the colon and rectum. It is characterized by inflammation confined to the mucosa (the most superficial layer) of the intestinal wall, but this inflammation can still be severe, causing deep ulceration in advanced cases. The disease always starts in the rectum and can spread continuously to the colon, but never affects the small intestine.

The main symptoms of ulcerative colitis are bloody diarrhea and rectorrhagia (discharge of blood from the anus), accompanied by abdominal pain, often localized in the lower abdomen. As with Crohn's disease, patients also suffer from severe fatigue, sometimes aggravated by blood loss leading to anemia. Outbreaks of ulcerative colitis can be violent, with frequent bloody diarrhoea, associated with intense abdominal pain and the urge to have a bowel movement (tenesmus). The disease also evolves in relapses and remissions, and its chronic nature requires regular medical monitoring.

Hemorrhagic rectocolitis can lead to a number of serious complications. One of the most dreaded is toxic megacolon, an acute, massive dilatation of the colon that can be life-threatening if not treated promptly. In addition, patients with long-term UC are at increased risk of developing colon cancer, which warrants regular endoscopic monitoring and biopsies to detect precancerous lesions.

Treatment of IBD

Treatment of IBD, whether Crohn's disease or ulcerative colitis, is based on a progressive approach aimed at controlling inflammation, relieving symptoms and preventing complications. Drug treatments generally include anti-inflammatories (such as mesalazine in the case of UC), immunosuppressants (such as azathioprine or methotrexate), and targeted biotherapies (such as TNF inhibitors like infliximab, or other molecules like ustekinumab). The latter have revolutionized the management of IBD, offering better chances of maintaining the disease in prolonged remission.

Treatment may also include corticosteroids to control acute flare-ups, but their long-term use is limited by numerous side effects, such as osteoporosis or diabetes. In some cases, particularly where there are complications such as fistulas, strictures or perforations, surgery becomes necessary. For patients with ulcerative colitis who do not respond to treatment, colectomy (total removal of the colon) can be a curative, albeit radical, option. Crohn's disease, on the other hand, being more diffuse, cannot be cured by surgery.

Impact on quality of life

IBD has a considerable impact on patients' quality of life, due not only to digestive symptoms, but also to systemic complications. These diseases are often associated with extra-intestinal manifestations, such as joint involvement (arthritis), skin lesions (erythema nodosum), or ocular inflammation (uveitis). Management of these conditions requires a multidisciplinary approach, involving not only the gastroenterologist, but also rheumatologists, dermatologists and ophthalmologists.

The chronic nature of these pathologies means that patients need close medical monitoring and constant adjustments to their treatment. Unpredictable relapses, drug side-effects and frequent surgery create great uncertainty and anxiety for patients. In addition, chronic fatigue, dietary restrictions, and repeated absences from work or school due to hospitalization or medical consultations make these diseases particularly disabling socially and professionally.

- Functional digestive disorders (irritable bowel syndrome, dyspepsia)

Functional digestive disorders, such as irritable bowel syndrome (IBS) and functional dyspepsia, are common but often poorly understood conditions. Unlike other digestive pathologies, which are characterized by visible structural abnormalities or inflammation, functional disorders generally reveal no identifiable organic lesions on endoscopic or radiological examination. However, they can cause very disabling symptoms, profoundly affecting patients' quality of life. These disorders mainly manifest themselves as abdominal pain, intestinal transit disorders, bloating or gastric burning sensations, with no specific underlying cause identifiable by conventional diagnostic methods.

Irritable bowel syndrome (IBS)

Irritable bowel syndrome, also known as functional colopathy, is one of the most common functional digestive disorders. It affects around 10-15% of the world's population, predominantly affecting young adults, with a higher prevalence in women. IBS is characterized by chronic abdominal pain associated with changes in intestinal transit, which may include diarrhea, constipation, or alternation between these two symptoms. These pains are often relieved by bowel movements, but their intensity and frequency vary from patient to patient.

The exact mechanism of IBS remains poorly understood, but several factors appear to contribute to its development. It is widely accepted that IBS results from a complex interaction between the brain-gut axis, intestinal motility, increased visceral sensitivity, and alterations in the intestinal flora (microbiota). This visceral sensitivity, which translates into an exaggerated reactivity of the intestines to normal stimuli such as gas or food digestion, is a central feature of IBS. Patients with this syndrome experience pain and discomfort at levels of intestinal pressure that would be tolerated without pain by individuals without IBS.

The role of stress and psychological factors is also crucial in IBS. Many patients report an exacerbation of their symptoms during periods of stress, anxiety or depression. This highlights the importance of the brain-gut axis in this pathology, where the central and enteric nervous systems communicate abnormally. Although IBS is an organically benign condition, the psychological and social impact can be considerable, with significant impairment of quality of life and consequences for social relationships, work and daily activities.

Functional dyspepsia

Functional dyspepsia, another major functional digestive disorder, manifests as localized pain or discomfort in the upper abdomen, often described as feelings of bloating, early satiety or heartburn. Like IBS, functional dyspepsia is not accompanied by any lesions visible on endoscopy or imaging, which can complicate diagnosis. This disorder is common, affecting around 20% of the world's population, although many people never consult a doctor for these symptoms.

Symptoms of functional dyspepsia can be triggered or exacerbated by food, particularly after eating rich, spicy or fatty meals. However, the role of food in this condition is not always clearly defined, and varies from one individual to another. Like IBS, patients with functional dyspepsia suffer from visceral hypersensitivity, where the stomach and intestine overreact to normal digestive processes. Disorders of gastrointestinal motility, such as delayed gastric emptying, may also play a role in the genesis of symptoms.

As with IBS, the psychological dimension is also an important factor in functional dyspepsia. Patients suffering from anxiety, chronic stress or depression are more likely to develop dyspepsia symptoms, and periods of emotional tension can aggravate sensations of gastric burning or heaviness. This link between functional disorders and emotions underlines the complexity of the pathology, where physiological and psychological mechanisms intertwine to create an altered perception of digestive sensations.

Management of functional digestive disorders

Treatment of functional digestive disorders, such as IBS and functional dyspepsia, is often multidimensional and focused on symptom relief, as there is no definitive cure. Management is generally based on a combination of lifestyle modifications, dietary changes and pharmacological treatments, with specific attention to psychological factors.

In the case of irritable bowel syndrome, diet plays a key role in managing symptoms. Many patients benefit from a specific dietary approach, such as the low FODMAP (Fermentable Oligo-, Di-, Mono-saccharides And Polyols) diet, which involves reducing consumption of certain fermentable carbohydrates. These foods, such as dairy products, certain fruits and vegetables, or legumes, can be poorly digested, leading to excessive gas production and an exacerbation of symptoms. In addition to these dietary measures, drug treatments can be used depending on the type of IBS. For example, laxatives are prescribed for constipating forms, and antidiarrheals for diarrheic forms. Antispasmodics and probiotics are also used to relieve abdominal pain and improve regulation of the intestinal microbiota.

Management of functional dyspepsia aims to reduce gastric symptoms through dietary adjustments (avoidance of heavy meals, fatty foods and carbonated beverages) and the use of medications such as antacids, proton pump inhibitors (PPIs) and prokinetics, which facilitate gastric emptying. However, the efficacy of drug treatments remains variable, and the therapeutic approach often needs to be tailored to the characteristics of the symptoms.

In both pathologies, the management of stress and psychological disorders is paramount. Approaches such as psychotherapy, cognitive-behavioural therapy (CBT) or relaxation can be of great help in reducing the impact of stress on digestive symptoms. Antidepressants, in low doses, are sometimes prescribed to modulate gut sensitivity and improve the patient's psychological state. This holistic approach is essential, as it addresses not only the physical symptoms, but also the underlying psychological factors that can exacerbate digestive disorders.

Impact on quality of life

Although functional digestive disorders are considered benign in terms of organic complications, they have a major impact on patients' quality of life. The recurrent and unpredictable symptoms, the anxiety associated with eating certain foods, and the social or professional embarrassment caused by abdominal pain or transit disorders create a real psychological burden. Many patients find it difficult to manage their daily life, their diet and their work, with significant repercussions on their emotional and relational well-being.

- Liver diseases (hepatitis, cirrhosis)

Liver pathologies, in particular hepatitis and cirrhosis, occupy a central place in gastroenterology because of their impact on the patient's overall health and the complexity of their management. The liver is an organ essential to the body's proper functioning, involved in such vital functions as blood detoxification, bile production, protein synthesis and nutrient storage. When this organ is impaired by chronic inflammation or progressive destruction of its cells, it has major systemic consequences, with repercussions not only on metabolism but also on other organs. Liver pathologies are often insidious, evolving silently for years before manifesting themselves through obvious symptoms, making them difficult to diagnose early and treat effectively.

Hepatitis

Hepatitis refers to inflammation of the liver and can be caused by a variety of factors, including viral infections (hepatitis A, B, C, D

44

and E), alcohol abuse, certain toxic substances (such as drugs or toxins), and autoimmune diseases. Viral hepatitis is one of the main causes of liver inflammation worldwide, and is responsible for millions of deaths every year.

Hepatitis A is generally contracted through consumption of contaminated food or water, and manifests itself through acute symptoms such as fever, jaundice, nausea and fatigue. It is often benign and heals spontaneously without sequelae, but can be serious in certain vulnerable populations. On the other hand, **hepatitis B and C can** develop into chronic forms, leading to serious complications such as cirrhosis and liver cancer. Hepatitis B is mainly transmitted by blood or sexual contact, while hepatitis C is mainly transmitted by contact with infected blood, notably during drug injections or unsafe blood transfusions.

Chronic forms of hepatitis B and C are particularly formidable, as they can evolve over many years without obvious symptoms, causing progressive destruction of liver tissue. Patients often only show signs when significant damage has already been done, in the form of jaundice, ascites (accumulation of fluid in the abdomen), or hepatic encephalopathy, resulting from an accumulation of toxins in the brain. Thanks to therapeutic advances, hepatitis C can now be cured with direct-acting antivirals, while hepatitis B can be controlled with antiviral treatments that prevent virus replication and slow disease progression.

Alcoholic hepatitis, on the other hand, is an inflammation of the liver caused by excessive and prolonged alcohol consumption. It can present in an acute form or evolve into chronic hepatitis, especially if alcohol consumption continues. Severe alcoholic hepatitis manifests itself through symptoms such as abdominal pain, jaundice and rapid weight loss. If left untreated, it can cause irreversible liver damage, leading to cirrhosis.

Cirrhosis

Cirrhosis is an advanced liver disease characterized by extensive fibrosis of the liver, resulting from the progressive destruction of liver cells and the formation of scar tissue. This scar tissue disrupts the normal structure of the liver, compromising its essential functions. Cirrhosis is often the consequence of untreated chronic hepatitis (viral hepatitis B or C) or excessive alcohol consumption over a long period. Other causes include metabolic diseases such as non-alcoholic fatty liver (NASH), which is associated with obesity, diabetes and metabolic syndrome.

The early stages of cirrhosis are often asymptomatic, making early diagnosis difficult. However, as the disease progresses, the liver gradually loses its ability to perform vital functions. Patients may then experience symptoms such as fatigue, weakness, loss of appetite and jaundice. Advanced cirrhosis can lead to serious complications, such as ascites (accumulation of fluid in the abdominal cavity), portal hypertension (increased blood pressure in the portal vein), esophageal varices that can rupture and cause digestive bleeding, and hepatic encephalopathy, a mental confusion caused by the liver's inability to eliminate toxins from the blood.

One of the most serious complications of cirrhosis is **hepatocellular carcinoma**, a liver cancer that often develops on a cirrhotic liver. The risk of developing liver cancer is particularly high in patients with chronic hepatitis B or C or alcoholic cirrhosis. The prognosis for this cancer is poor when diagnosed at an advanced stage, underlining the importance of regular screening of patients with cirrhosis, through ultrasound scans and alpha-fetoprotein (a tumor marker) assays.

Management of liver diseases

The management of liver disease varies according to the underlying cause, the stage of the disease and the presence of complications. For viral hepatitis B and C, antiviral treatment is the cornerstone of disease management. Today, hepatitis C patients benefit from highly effective curative treatments, while hepatitis B requires lifelong treatment to control replication of the virus. Vaccination against hepatitis B is also a crucial preventive measure to reduce the incidence of this infection.

In the case of **cirrhosis**, treatment is aimed at slowing disease progression and preventing complications. This may include diuretics to manage ascites, beta-blockers to reduce the risk of variceal haemorrhage, and treatments to prevent hepatic encephalopathy. Cessation of alcohol consumption is paramount for patients with alcoholic cirrhosis, and withdrawal programs can be offered to help patients overcome their dependence.

Liver transplantation remains the treatment of last resort for patients with decompensated cirrhosis or end-stage liver cancer. The procedure, although complex, offers a chance of long-term survival for patients whose livers can no longer function. However, the shortage of grafts and strict selection criteria limit access to this option for many patients.

Impact of liver disease on quality of life

Liver disease, particularly when it progresses to cirrhosis, has a devastating impact on patients' quality of life. Chronic fatigue, fluid accumulation in the abdomen, and mental confusion make daily life difficult to manage. In addition, dietary restrictions, complex treatment management, and frequent hospitalizations to treat complications increase the emotional and physical burden. Patients suffering from decompensated cirrhosis often require constant support, and families are often involved in long-term care, which can weigh heavily on those around them.

- Digestive tumors (colon, stomach, liver cancers)

Digestive tract tumors, particularly cancers of the colon, stomach and liver, constitute a group of serious and potentially fatal pathologies that affect a large proportion of the world's population. They represent a major challenge in gastroenterology, due to their growing incidence and the challenges posed by their early diagnosis, treatment and follow-up. These cancers are often insidious, developing slowly over several years before being detected, which complicates their management. Despite therapeutic advances and screening campaigns, these pathologies remain one of the world's leading causes of mortality. Their management requires a multidisciplinary approach involving gastroenterologists, surgeons, oncologists and radiologists, with treatment strategies combining surgery, chemotherapy, radiotherapy and, in some cases, immunotherapy.

Colon cancer

Colon cancer, or colorectal cancer, is one of the most common digestive cancers worldwide, particularly in industrialized countries. It mainly affects people over the age of 50, but can also affect younger individuals, especially in the presence of genetic predispositions such as familial adenomatous polyposis (FAP) or Lynch syndrome. The development of colon cancer is often linked to the malignant transformation of adenomatous polyps present in the colonic mucosa. This transformation can take several years, providing a valuable opportunity for early detection and intervention.

Systematic screening by colonoscopy is an essential weapon in reducing mortality from colon cancer. By identifying and removing polyps before they develop into cancer, many cases can be prevented. Screening programs generally recommend surveillance colonoscopy from the age of 50, or even earlier in people with a family history of colorectal cancer, or predisposing diseases such as chronic inflammatory bowel disease (Crohn's disease, ulcerative colitis).

The early stages of colon cancer are often asymptomatic, which is why screening is crucial. When symptoms do appear, they may include abdominal pain, changes in bowel transit (constipation or diarrhea), blood in the stool, unexplained anemia, or weight loss. At an advanced stage, the cancer can cause intestinal obstruction, necessitating emergency surgery. The mainstay of treatment is surgery to remove the affected portion of the colon (colectomy). This surgery is often combined with adjuvant chemotherapy to reduce the risk of recurrence, particularly if the cancer is detected at an advanced stage or if lymph nodes are involved.

Stomach cancer

Stomach cancer, or gastric cancer, is less common than colon cancer, but remains one of the leading causes of cancer deaths worldwide, particularly in East Asia. This cancer generally develops from the lining of the stomach and can take several forms, the most common of which is adenocarcinoma. Risk factors include infection with *Helicobacter pylori* (a bacterium responsible for gastric ulcers), smoking, alcohol, as well as dietary factors such as a diet rich in salt and smoked foods. Genetic predisposition also exists, notably in cases of familial gastric cancer.

Stomach cancer is often diagnosed late, because the early symptoms are vague and non-specific, such as epigastric pain, heartburn, early satiety or loss of appetite. These symptoms are often confused with those of functional dyspepsia or a simple gastric ulcer, delaying diagnosis. When cancer reaches a more advanced stage, it may cause digestive bleeding, marked weight loss, or recurrent vomiting. A late sign is the presence of palpable lymph nodes in the clavicle (Troisier lymph node), often indicating metastatic spread.

Treatment of stomach cancer relies mainly on surgery, which involves removal of all or part of the stomach (gastrectomy), depending on the location and extent of the tumour. Chemotherapy and radiotherapy are often combined to improve chances of survival, especially in advanced stages. Immunotherapy has also shown promising results in some cases, particularly for cancers expressing specific markers such as

49

HER2. However, the prognosis of gastric cancer remains guarded, especially if detected late, hence the importance of early detection in at-risk populations, particularly those exposed to *Helicobacter pylori*.

Liver cancer

Liver cancer, or hepatocellular carcinoma (HCC), is one of the most aggressive digestive tumors, often associated with underlying cirrhosis. The main causes of this cancer are chronic infection with the hepatitis B and C viruses, as well as chronic alcoholism and non-alcoholic fatty liver disease (NASH), the latter being increasingly common due to the rise in obesity and type 2 diabetes worldwide. Cirrhosis, whatever its etiology, is a major risk factor for the development of liver cancer, as the progressive destruction of liver tissue favours the appearance of tumours.

Liver cancer is often silent in its early stages, but signs such as unexplained weight loss, pain in the right hypochondrium, jaundice, or the appearance of a distended abdomen due to ascites can signal advanced disease. Regular screening of cirrhotic patients, via liver ultrasound and alpha-fetoprotein blood tests, is therefore essential for early detection of hepatocellular carcinoma.

Treatment of liver cancer depends on a number of factors, including the size and number of tumors, remaining liver function, and the extent of the disease. Treatment options include surgical resection (in cases where the tumor is isolated and the patient has good liver function), liver transplantation (for patients with multiple tumors or decompensated cirrhosis), and local treatments such as radiofrequency or chemoembolization, which aim to reduce tumor size. In more advanced stages, systemic treatments such as sorafenib (a tyrosine kinase inhibitor) or immunotherapy are used, although the prognosis often remains poor when cancer is detected late.

Multidisciplinary management and prevention

The management of digestive tumors, whether colon, stomach or liver cancers, requires a multidisciplinary approach. Gastroenterologists, digestive surgeons, oncologists, radiologists and pathologists work together to establish the diagnosis and propose the best treatment strategy. Decisions are often taken at multidisciplinary concertation meetings (RCP), where the specifics of each case are discussed, taking into account the patient's general condition, the characteristics of the tumor and the treatment options available.

Prevention plays a key role in the fight against digestive cancers. For colon cancer, screening by colonoscopy is a highly effective measure, enabling polyps to be detected and removed before they become cancerous. For stomach cancer, prevention involves eradicating *Helicobacter pylori* infection in at-risk populations. Finally, for liver cancer, vaccination against hepatitis B, treatment of hepatitis C, and the fight against alcoholism and obesity are essential preventive measures.

- Biliary and pancreatic disorders

Biliary and pancreatic diseases are a key area of gastroenterology, due to their often severe impact on patient health and the complexity of their management. These pathologies concern essential organs of the digestive system: the gallbladder, the bile ducts and the pancreas. They include common conditions such as biliary lithiasis, and more serious and sometimes fatal diseases such as pancreatic cancer or acute pancreatitis. The diversity of biliary and pancreatic disorders requires multidisciplinary and often urgent management, due to the acute nature of some complications and the systemic impact of these conditions on metabolism and digestion.

Biliary disorders

Biliary disorders mainly affect the gallbladder and bile ducts, which play an essential role in the storage and transport of bile, a liquid produced by the liver to help digest fats. Bile is stored in the gallbladder and released into the small intestine after meals to aid digestion. When this process is disrupted, due to gallstones or other abnormalities, severe pain and complications can occur.

Biliary lithiasis, or gallstones, is one of the most common biliary disorders. It is characterized by the formation of solid crystals, often cholesterol-based, in the gallbladder. These stones can remain asymptomatic for years, or cause biliary colic, intense pain in the right hypochondrium, especially after high-fat meals. In some cases, these stones can migrate into the bile ducts, leading to serious complications such as acute cholecystitis (inflammation of the gallbladder), angiocholitis (infection of the bile ducts), or acute pancreatitis. These complications require prompt management, often through surgery to remove the gallbladder (cholecystectomy) or endoscopic surgery (ERCP) to extract stones obstructing the bile ducts.

Acute cholecystitis, which generally results from obstruction of the cystic duct by a stone, is an inflammation of the gallbladder. It manifests as severe abdominal pain, fever and general malaise. If not treated promptly, cholecystitis can progress to more serious complications, such as gallbladder perforation or peritonitis. Treatment of acute cholecystitis often involves emergency surgery to remove the gallbladder, accompanied by antibiotic therapy to treat the infection.

Angiocholitis, also known as cholangitis, is an infection of the bile ducts that occurs when these are obstructed by a stone or tumor. The condition manifests itself as the classic Charcot triad of abdominal pain, fever and jaundice. Angiocholitis is a medical emergency, as the infection can rapidly spread throughout the body, leading to septic shock. Treatment relies on rapid decompression of the bile ducts, often by endoscopy (ERCP), to remove the obstruction, and aggressive antibiotic therapy to eradicate the infection.

Pancreatic disorders

Pancreatic disorders are often serious and require rapid, specialized treatment. The pancreas is an essential organ for digestion and blood sugar regulation. It secretes digestive enzymes that help break down fats, proteins and carbohydrates, as well as hormones, such as insulin, that regulate sugar metabolism. When the pancreas is affected by inflammation or tumor, this can lead to serious consequences, from intense abdominal pain to pancreatic insufficiency and diabetes.

Acute pancreatitis is one of the most urgent pancreatic disorders. It is generally caused by obstruction of the pancreatic duct by a gallstone, or by excessive alcohol consumption. Acute pancreatitis is characterized by sudden inflammation of the pancreas, with intense abdominal pain often radiating to the back, nausea and vomiting. In severe forms, acute pancreatitis can lead to systemic complications such as respiratory failure, renal failure or septic shock. Treatment involves emergency hospitalization, with intensive medical support including rehydration, pain management, and sometimes surgery to remove gallstones or drain fluid collections around the pancreas. In some cases, acute pancreatitis may progress to pancreatic necrosis, requiring surgical or endoscopic intervention to remove the necrotic tissue.

Chronic pancreatitis is an inflammation of the pancreas that evolves over several years, leading to progressive destruction of pancreatic tissue. It is often linked to excessive and prolonged alcohol consumption, although other causes, such as congenital abnormalities of the pancreatic ducts, autoimmune diseases or genetic factors, may also be involved. Chronic pancreatitis causes recurrent abdominal pain, exocrine pancreatic insufficiency (inability to digest food properly), and, in advanced stages, endocrine pancreatic insufficiency (diabetes). Treatment is aimed at relieving pain, replacing missing pancreatic enzymes with supplements, and preventing complications. In some cases, surgery may be required to treat complications such as stenosis of the pancreatic duct or pseudocysts.

Pancreatic cancer is one of the most aggressive and difficult tumors to treat. It is often diagnosed at an advanced stage due to the absence of early symptoms. Symptoms, when they appear, include abdominal pain, weight loss, jaundice (when the tumor obstructs the bile duct), and sometimes digestive disorders. Pancreatic cancer has a dismal prognosis, with a very low five-year survival rate, largely due to the difficulty of diagnosing it early and resistance to treatment. Treatment relies on surgery, but only a minority of tumors are resectable at the time of diagnosis. Chemotherapy and, in some cases, radiotherapy are used to prolong survival, but results are often limited. Current research is focusing on new approaches, such as immunotherapy, to improve the chances of survival for patients suffering from this pathology.

Management of biliary and pancreatic diseases

The management of biliary and pancreatic diseases requires a multidisciplinary approach, involving gastroenterologists, surgeons, radiologists and oncologists. In the case of biliary disorders, endoscopic procedures play a central role in treating stones and draining the bile ducts. For pancreatic disorders, treatment can range from intensive medical care for acute pancreatitis to surgery for pancreatic tumors. Pain management, correction of nutritional deficits, and treatment of complications are essential elements of long-term management, particularly in chronic pancreatitis.

Impact on quality of life

Biliary and pancreatic disorders, particularly in their acute or severe forms, have a major impact on patients' quality of life. Recurrent abdominal pain, frequent hospitalizations, and the need to follow a strict diet or take enzyme supplements make daily life difficult to manage for many patients. What's more, pancreatic disorders, when they lead to exocrine or endocrine pancreatic insufficiency, require ongoing adaptation of management, notably with replacement treatments and close monitoring to prevent complications.

3 The impact of these pathologies on the patient and the role of the caregiver

*   Impaired quality of life

Impaired quality of life is a major consequence of digestive disease, whether acute or chronic, benign or severe. It is an essential dimension of patient care, because beyond the physical symptoms, the repercussions on daily life, social relationships and mental health are often profound and long-lasting. The impact of gastrointestinal pathologies is not limited to pain or physical discomfort. These illnesses affect a person's overall balance, modifying their relationship with food, their body, their loved ones, and their professional or social environment.

Symptoms and their impact on daily life

The symptoms associated with digestive diseases can be extremely disabling, even when they are not immediately life-threatening. Chronic abdominal pain, diarrhea, constipation, vomiting or bloating disrupt patients' daily lives, making it difficult to perform simple tasks and social interactions. In conditions such as irritable bowel syndrome (IBS) or chronic inflammatory bowel disease (IBD), these symptoms are unpredictable, adding to the stress and uncertainty for patients. They often have to adjust their schedules, avoid certain foods, and live with the constant fear of a relapse or flare-up of symptoms.

Daily management of symptoms often involves strict dietary adjustments, regular medication, and even invasive treatments such as infusions or injections for patients with chronic diseases. These constraints weigh heavily on patients, who may feel restricted in their dietary, social and even professional choices.

Meals, a central moment in social life, often become a source of anxiety. People with digestive disorders may fear eating in public, being confronted with trigger foods, or having to manage uncomfortable symptoms in social or professional situations.

Psychological repercussions

Chronic digestive diseases have a profound effect on patients' mental health. Constant pain and discomfort, combined with uncertainty about the course of the disease, are major factors in anxiety and depression. In pathologies such as Crohn's disease or ulcerative colitis, where inflammatory flare-ups can occur unpredictably, anticipatory anxiety becomes frequent: patients dread each new crisis and live in fear of having to be hospitalized or undergo surgery.

The feeling of losing control over one's body, dependence on medication, and sometimes the need for permanent medical devices, such as an ostomy, reinforce this malaise. Patients may also feel that their body image is devalued, and that they are stigmatized or isolated. This psychological dimension is often underestimated, but it plays a crucial role in how patients perceive their disease and their overall quality of life. Digestive disorders are particularly intimate, touching on such personal aspects as digestion, eating and elimination - functions that are often taboo in society. Feelings of shame or embarrassment can lead to social isolation, with a reluctance to share difficulties, even with loved ones.

Impact on social and family relations

The loss of quality of life associated with digestive disease also extends to social and family relationships. Patients suffering from chronic or recurrent illnesses can feel like a burden to those around them. Repeated absences from work or social activities, frequent hospitalizations, and the inability to participate in events or meals can create a gulf between patients and their loved ones. The latter, while often understanding, may also feel powerless in the face of the sick person's suffering, or overwhelmed by the burden of having to constantly adapt to their loved one's state of health.

Intimate relationships may also be affected, due to fatigue, chronic pain or altered body image. People with digestive diseases may experience a loss of sexual desire or discomfort linked to their condition, which can create tension in couples. Psychological support and open communication are essential to help overcome these relationship difficulties, but the fact remains that these diseases impose an emotional and physical burden that profoundly affects relationship dynamics.

Professional impact

At work, digestive disorders can lead to frequent absences, prolonged work stoppages and reduced performance. Patients suffering from chronic disorders often have to juggle medical treatment, regular consultations and the day-to-day management of their symptoms, which can prevent them from leading a stable working life. In some cases, people have to consider a career change or part-time work due to the inability to maintain a steady work pace.

This professional instability can lead to financial difficulties, further exacerbating the impact of the disease on quality of life. In addition, patients may feel that they are not understood or supported by their employers and colleagues, especially when symptoms are not visible or the disease is not well known to the general public. This feeling of being misunderstood and marginalized can increase patients' isolation and sense of social exclusion.

Long-term disease management

For patients suffering from chronic digestive diseases, managing their disease can be a long and arduous process. The need for regular medical monitoring, lifelong treatment or frequent changes in treatment protocols creates a sense of fatigue and weariness. The constant need to watch one's diet, take medication and cope with relapses takes its toll on patients' morale. The idea of living with a disease that cannot be cured, but only controlled, can provoke feelings of helplessness and frustration.

In this context, medical, psychological and social support is crucial. A multidisciplinary approach, including not only gastroenterologists, but also psychologists, dieticians and patient associations, can help to better manage the impact of the disease on quality of life. Stress management strategies, behavioral and cognitive therapies, and support for family and friends are essential to help patients live better with their disease.

• Specific patient needs: physical and psychological aspects
The specific needs of patients with digestive diseases, whether acute or chronic, are numerous and complex. These needs go beyond the simple management of physical symptoms, and touch on fundamental aspects of daily physical, psychological and social life. These patients face an altered quality of life, often burdensome and restrictive treatments, and emotional challenges linked to the uncertainty of their condition. A holistic approach to their care, which takes account of these different dimensions, is essential if they are to receive appropriate, personalized support.

Physical aspects: relieving symptoms and improving comfort

The physical symptoms of digestive diseases are often severe and recurrent, imposing specific needs that vary according to the pathology, its stage of progression, and the patient's general condition. Pain is a ubiquitous symptom in many digestive diseases, from biliary colic and abdominal pain in irritable bowel syndrome, to cramps associated with chronic inflammatory bowel disease. Managing this pain is a priority, as it disrupts not only the patient's comfort, but also his or her ability to lead a normal life. The need for pain relief can be met by appropriate drug treatments, such as antispasmodics or analgesics, but also by non-drug approaches, such as relaxation, stress management techniques, or personalized diets that reduce the triggers for attacks.

In addition to pain, intestinal transit disorders - diarrhea, constipation, bloating - are frequent sources of discomfort for patients. These symptoms not only cause physical discomfort, but also a social handicap, as patients often have to adjust their lifestyle and movements to the frequency of these symptoms. It is essential to adapt treatments to normalize transit, combining specific dietary advice, probiotics and drugs to regulate intestinal motility. Caregivers and nurses play a key role in supporting patients, identifying when additional interventions are needed and proposing strategies to minimize the impact of these disorders on daily life.

Patients suffering from chronic diseases, such as Crohn's disease or cirrhosis, have specific nutritional needs. Malabsorption of nutrients is common in these pathologies, leading to deficiencies that require supplementation and regular monitoring. Dieticians are often involved in devising adapted diets, aimed at limiting symptom exacerbations while ensuring adequate nutritional intake. For some patients, enteral or parenteral nutrition may be necessary, particularly in the acute phases of the disease, when the intestine can no longer ensure proper digestion. Nutritional management then becomes an essential part of the treatment, requiring close monitoring to avoid undernutrition and maintain the patient's strength.

Psychological aspects: dealing with anxiety, depression and uncertainty

Psychologically, the needs of patients suffering from digestive diseases are just as crucial, but often underestimated. Digestive diseases, particularly chronic pathologies such as IBD or digestive cancers, profoundly affect patients' emotional and mental well-being. Anxiety is one of the most common psychological disorders in these patients, fuelled by the unpredictability of symptoms, the fear of flare-ups or recurrences, and the anguish associated with frequent medical interventions. Not knowing when another attack will occur, or the idea of having to undergo another operation or hospitalization, creates constant insecurity. Patients can experience intense stress that worsens digestive symptoms, fuelling a vicious circle between body and mind.

Depression is also common, especially in patients facing serious illnesses such as cancer or cirrhosis, where the prognosis may be uncertain or bleak. The feeling of losing control over one's body, chronic fatigue, and the limitations imposed by the disease, such as dietary restrictions or work absences, can lead to a sense of helplessness, even despair. This psychological malaise is often compounded by the loneliness and social isolation these illnesses engender. It is not uncommon for patients to feel misunderstood by those around them, who do not always perceive the extent of their suffering or the difficulty of living with an invisible disease.

Given these psychological needs, psychological support must be an essential component of care. This can include the intervention of psychologists or psychiatrists specialized in chronic diseases, as well as behavioral and cognitive therapies, which help patients to better manage their stress and anxiety. Talking groups and patient associations can also provide valuable support, enabling patients to share their experiences and break down social isolation. By being in direct and regular contact with patients, caregivers play a key role in detecting signs of psychological distress and can alert the medical team to offer appropriate support.

Uncertainty as to how the disease will progress is another source of anxiety for patients, particularly those with digestive cancers or chronic progressive pathologies such as cirrhosis. The fear of relapse, the fear of a rapid deterioration in health, or the anxiety linked to heavy treatments such as chemotherapy or liver transplantation, are all stress factors that weigh heavily on patients' morale. In such cases, it is crucial to provide clear, regular information on the progress of the disease, available treatments and future prospects, while remaining attentive to patients' fears and questions. Transparency and benevolent communication are essential to allaying concerns and reinforcing the patient's sense of security.

The need for relational and social support

In addition to the physical and psychological aspects, patients with digestive diseases have a crucial need for relational and social support. The disease, especially when chronic, profoundly alters family, friends and professional relationships. Patients need an understanding and caring family and friends, able to support them in difficult times and accompany them through the various stages of their care. Relatives often have to adapt to the constraints imposed by the disease, whether by adjusting meals, accompanying the patient to medical consultations, or offering moral support in times of doubt or discouragement.

However, this support is not always easy to find. Some patients may feel like a burden to their loved ones, especially when the disease requires constant attention. Others may isolate themselves for fear of being disturbed or not understood. It is therefore important for healthcare teams to encourage open dialogue between patients and those around them, and to provide tools to help families better understand the disease and better support their loved ones.

Chapter 2

The role of the gastroenterology orderly: multiple skills

1 The caregiver's main missions

• Assisting patients with daily care (hygiene, comfort)
Supporting patients in their daily care, whether in terms of hygiene or comfort, is an essential component of gastroenterology care, particularly for those suffering from chronic or serious pathologies. This daily support, largely provided by nursing aides, plays a fundamental role in patients' physical and psychological well-being. Over and above medical care, the aim is to ensure that each patient retains his or her dignity, comfort and acceptable quality of life, despite the constraints imposed by the disease. This daily care, which may seem simple, is in fact of crucial importance in helping patients to live better with their condition, by providing them with a sense of security and care.

Hygiene care: an act of dignity and comfort

Personal hygiene is a central aspect of daily care, particularly for patients who are hospitalized or bedridden due to their illness. In a gastroenterology department, patients may be confronted with symptoms such as diarrhea, vomiting, or skin conditions linked to pathologies such as fistulas or stomas. These situations, often a source of discomfort, require special attention. The caregiver intervenes to ensure that body hygiene is maintained in the best possible conditions, taking care to clean, protect and moisturize the patient's skin, to prevent infection or irritation.

Hygiene care, beyond its technical aspect, is also a time for exchange and humanity. For patients who are losing their autonomy, sometimes unable to move about on their own or to go to the toilet, being helped with these intimate gestures can be a source of embarrassment or vulnerability. It is therefore crucial for the caregiver to demonstrate great benevolence, empathy and discretion, so that these moments of care are experienced as serenely as possible. By maintaining the patient's dignity, the caregiver plays an active role in his or her psychological well-being. This involves simple gestures: explaining each stage of care, respecting modesty by using sheets to cover parts of the body not involved in care, and adapting to the patient's needs and preferences.

For patients with medical devices such as nasogastric tubes, catheters or stomas, hygiene must be particularly rigorous. This means keeping these devices clean, avoiding maceration or irritation, and regularly checking for signs of infection. The caregiver plays a key role here, monitoring the condition of these devices on a daily basis and ensuring that the patient is comfortable with their care. In the case of ostomies, for example, support in managing the pouch is essential. The patient must learn how to change the pouch, clean the skin around the stoma and recognize the signs of possible complications. In addition to performing these tasks, the caregiver plays an educational role, explaining best practices and reassuring the patient about a situation that can be difficult to accept.

Physical and emotional comfort: a pillar of quality of life

Patient comfort is another fundamental aspect of daily care. In the context of digestive disease, where abdominal pain, bloating and nausea are frequent, the caregiver must ensure that each patient is installed comfortably, to minimize the discomfort associated with his or her condition. This can include simple gestures such as adjusting the bed's inclination, offering cushions to support certain parts of the body, or ensuring proper hydration. A patient confined to bed for long periods of time can quickly suffer from pain linked to poor posture, or develop bedsores. The caregiver must therefore ensure regular mobilization to prevent these complications and guarantee a comfortable position.

Patient comfort also involves managing body temperature. Patients, especially those suffering from fever or severe digestive disorders, may feel hot or cold. Ensuring that they are properly covered or, on the contrary, cooled, provides them with a more pleasant environment, conducive to rest and recuperation. What's more, by providing them with a clean, orderly care environment adapted to their needs (particularly in terms of lighting and noise), the caregiver helps to create a soothing environment.

Emotional comfort is also a central issue. Patients suffering from chronic or severe digestive diseases are often anxious, troubled by unpredictable symptoms and heavy treatments. They may feel frustrated by their loss of autonomy, or fearful about the future course of their disease. At such times, the caregiver's constant, reassuring presence can provide invaluable support. A simple attentive listening ear, a reassuring word, or a clear explanation of the course of care can allay the patient's anxieties. The caregiver then becomes a reference point, a trusted person to whom the patient can confide his or her worries or discomforts.

Patient empowerment and moral support

Another important aspect of daily care support is the gradual empowerment of the patient, wherever possible. The aim is to encourage patients to actively participate in their own care, according to their abilities. This can start with simple gestures, such as washing hands, taking part in toileting, or learning to manage medical devices. By involving the patient in these gestures, the caregiver fosters a sense of control over the disease, which can be particularly beneficial for morale. Indeed, loss of autonomy can be experienced as an attack on personal dignity, and every gesture a patient can perform alone represents a victory over the disease.

For patients at the end of life, or in the terminal phase of a serious illness, support in daily care takes on a special dimension. The aim is to maintain the patient's comfort at all times, by relieving pain, preventing bedsores and respecting the patient's wishes as far as possible. The caregiver's role at this time is also to support the family, by explaining the care provided and creating a soothing, respectful environment for all concerned.

- Monitoring of clinical signs (vomiting, diarrhea, abdominal pain)

Monitoring clinical signs such as vomiting, diarrhea and abdominal pain is a fundamental aspect of gastroenterology patient management. These symptoms, frequent in digestive diseases, are not only a source of suffering for the patient, but can also be indicators of worsening health or underlying complications. Rigorous and continuous observation of clinical signs enables us to anticipate deterioration, react rapidly and adapt treatments accordingly. For the care team, this constant vigilance is essential to ensure patient safety, prevent potentially serious complications, and guarantee optimal care.

Vomiting: a sign to watch out for

Vomiting, whether isolated or recurrent, is a frequent symptom of gastrointestinal pathologies. It can be linked to functional digestive disorders, infections, intestinal obstructions or more serious conditions such as pancreatitis, gastric ulcers or digestive tumors. Monitoring vomiting is therefore crucial to identifying the underlying cause and assessing the severity of the problem.

When vomiting occurs, several parameters need to be observed. Firstly, the frequency and duration of vomiting give an indication of the intensity of the problem. Frequent and repeated vomiting can rapidly lead to severe dehydration, especially in vulnerable patients such as the elderly or children. It is therefore essential to watch for signs of dehydration, such as dry mouth, reduced diuresis, fatigue or confusion. In this context, oral or intravenous hydration may be necessary to compensate for fluid losses.

The nature of the vomiting should also be carefully considered. Vomiting containing traces of blood (hematemesis) may indicate upper GI bleeding, potentially linked to gastric ulcer or esophageal varices. This clinical sign requires emergency treatment. Similarly, dark green, bile-like vomiting may indicate intestinal obstruction, especially if associated with abdominal pain and an absence of stool or gas. In this case, urgent surgical intervention may be considered.

Finally, the management of vomiting involves rapid relief of the patient's symptoms. In addition to monitoring, the nursing team must provide appropriate antiemetic treatments to stop or limit episodes of vomiting, while keeping the patient in a comfortable, secure position to avoid the risk of inhalation, particularly in weakened patients.

Diarrhea: a sign with many causes

Diarrhea is another common symptom in gastroenterology, and its monitoring is of paramount importance. Diarrhea can be caused by gastrointestinal infections, chronic inflammatory bowel disease (such as Crohn's disease or ulcerative colitis), food intolerances, or the side effects of medication. Acute diarrhea can rapidly lead to dehydration and electrolyte imbalance, especially if it is abundant and prolonged. Careful monitoring of stool frequency, volume and appearance is therefore essential.

When a patient presents with diarrhea, it's important to observe several aspects. Firstly, the frequency of bowel movements: persistent diarrhea with frequent, watery stools should alert you to the risk of dehydration. The health-care team should watch for associated signs, such as hypotension, increased heart rate or lethargy, which indicate a state of dehydration requiring rapid intervention, either orally or intravenously.

The appearance of stools is also a key indicator. Stools containing blood (rectorrhagia) or mucus, particularly in the case of inflammatory bowel disease, may indicate a relapse of the disease, necessitating a reassessment of treatment. Pale, fatty or steatorrhea-like stools may indicate malabsorption linked to pancreatic or biliary disorders. In such cases, specific nutritional and medical management is required.

Managing diarrhea involves not only monitoring clinical parameters, but also symptomatic management to improve patient comfort. Anti-diarrhoeal drugs may be prescribed, depending on the underlying cause, but it is equally important to ensure hydration and electrolyte rebalancing, particularly in at-risk patients such as the elderly or immunocompromised.

Abdominal pain: a complex and revealing symptom

Abdominal pain is another central symptom of digestive disease, and can have multiple causes. Whether acute or chronic, monitoring abdominal pain is essential for orienting diagnosis and adapting management. The location, intensity, duration and triggers or relievers of pain provide valuable clues as to the nature of the underlying problem.

Acute abdominal pain, especially if severe and associated with vomiting or fever, can reveal serious pathologies, such as appendicitis, intestinal obstruction, acute pancreatitis or perforation of a digestive organ. In these situations, the health-care team must react quickly to carry out additional tests (medical imaging, blood tests) and determine the need for emergency surgery. Patients suffering from acute pain should be closely monitored for signs of aggravation, such as abdominal rigidity, signs of shock (hypotension, tachycardia), or rapid deterioration in general condition.

Chronic abdominal pain, often present in pathologies such as irritable bowel syndrome or chronic inflammatory bowel disease, also requires careful monitoring. Although often less severe than acute pain, it can significantly impair patients' quality of life. The caregiver must listen carefully to the patient to identify when pain is increasing, and the factors that relieve it (change of position, taking medication) or aggravate it (food intake, stress). This vigilance enables them to adjust treatments, whether antispasmodics, analgesics or dietary modifications, to improve patient comfort.

69

The caregiver's role in clinical monitoring

Caregivers play a vital role in monitoring clinical signs. By being in constant contact with the patient, they can observe the evolution of symptoms on a daily basis, whether vomiting, diarrhea or abdominal pain. This monitoring role enables the medical team to be alerted rapidly in the event of a change in symptoms, a deterioration in general condition, or the appearance of new signs. The nursing auxiliary is also on the front line in gathering patient complaints, assessing the effectiveness of symptomatic treatments, and adjusting care to improve comfort and prevent complications.

- Assistance with gastroenterological examinations and procedures

Assisting with gastroenterological examinations and procedures is a crucial task requiring close collaboration between nursing aides, nurses and gastroenterologists. These examinations, such as colonoscopy, gastroscopy and other endoscopic procedures, as well as interventions such as catheterization and biopsies, play a central role in the diagnosis, treatment and monitoring of digestive pathologies. The nursing auxiliary plays a key role in this process, ensuring not only the technical preparation of patients and equipment, but also their comfort and safety, and the management of the immediate aftermath of interventions.

Patient preparation: ensuring serenity and comfort

The first step in assisting with gastroenterological examinations is to prepare the patient both physically and mentally. These examinations can be a source of anxiety for many patients, who are often apprehensive about physical discomfort or the diagnostic result. The nursing auxiliary is therefore there to reassure the patient, explain the procedure simply and clearly, and answer any questions or fears. This human dimension is essential, as it helps to reduce the patient's anxiety, thus ensuring that the examination goes smoothly.

On the physical side, patient preparation can include several steps, depending on the type of procedure. For a colonoscopy, for example, the patient must follow a specific diet and take laxatives the day before the examination to cleanse the bowel. The caregiver ensures that these instructions are followed, while making sure that the patient is well hydrated and ready for the examination. They also help to position the patient on the examination table in a suitable position, often lying on the left side, to facilitate insertion of the endoscope. This is a crucial moment to ensure patient comfort and prevent unnecessary stress.

Technical assistance during examinations

During the examination itself, the nursing auxiliary plays a technical assistance role, providing direct support to the gastroenterologist and the nurse. One of their main tasks is to ensure that the medical equipment is in good working order, that everything is ready for the procedure, and to respond rapidly to the doctor's needs throughout the procedure. This includes preparing endoscopes, checking monitoring equipment (such as pulse oximeters or blood pressure monitors to monitor vital signs), and managing suction devices to remove secretions that could impede visualization of digestive structures.

As part of an endoscopy (whether colonoscopy or gastroscopy), the caregiver may also be called upon to support the patient during the examination, in particular by helping him or her to maintain an appropriate position, or by encouraging the patient to remain calm and relaxed. In the case of light sedation, the caregiver must carefully monitor the patient's signs of comfort or discomfort, and report any signs of abnormality to the doctor or nurse. Their proximity to the patient enables them to be particularly attentive to immediate needs, such as adjusting an uncomfortable position, offering a towel to wipe secretions, or simply reassuring the patient with a caring presence.

Support in therapeutic interventions

In addition to diagnostic examinations, many gastroenterological procedures are therapeutic in nature. These may include the removal of polyps during a colonoscopy, the dilatation of a stenosis (narrowing of a digestive passage), or the placement of stents in obstructed bile ducts. The caregiver's assistance is just as essential here, as these procedures are often more complex and require perfect coordination between the medical and paramedical teams.

The nursing auxiliary ensures that the necessary instruments, such as biopsy forceps, catheters and dilatation balloons, are readily available and perfectly sterilized. In addition, depending on the complexity of the procedure, the orderly may be asked to monitor the patient's vital signs more closely, in collaboration with the nurse, particularly if deep sedation or anesthesia is required. These procedures can last longer than a simple examination, and maintaining the patient's comfort and safety remains a priority.

Management of the immediate aftermath of the examination or procedure

Once the examination or procedure has been completed, the nursing auxiliary's role continues in the immediate aftermath. They help the patient recover from the examination, particularly if sedation has been administered. This includes monitoring residual effects of sedation, such as drowsiness or dizziness, and helping the patient return to the room or rest area. The caregiver also ensures that the patient is comfortable and reassured, explaining that side effects such as bloating or slight discomfort are normal after certain examinations, such as a colonoscopy.

Observing clinical signs in the hours following a procedure is crucial. In particular, the caregiver looks out for signs of complications, such as severe pain, vomiting, bleeding or low blood pressure, which could indicate intestinal perforation or digestive bleeding. If these signs appear, the caregiver must immediately alert the medical team for rapid treatment. This careful monitoring helps to prevent serious complications, and ensures continuous patient surveillance.

Finally, the caregiver plays a key role in educating the patient about post-procedure care. Whether after nasogastric tube placement, biliary stenting or polyp resection, they must provide clear information on precautions to take, warning signs to watch out for, and dietary or medication recommendations. This educational dimension is essential to ensure a safe recovery and avoid complications at home.

2 Working with the multidisciplinary team

• The caregiver's role in transmitting information
The caregiver's role in transmitting information is fundamental to the smooth running of any care team. In gastroenterology, where patients often suffer from complex and progressive pathologies, this transmission of information takes on particular importance. The nursing auxiliary, in direct and constant contact with the patient, plays a key role in observing clinical signs, communicating changes in the patient's state of health, and passing on essential information to other members of the medical team. This effective communication guarantees optimal, rapid and appropriate care, while ensuring continuity of care. The caregiver's role is therefore not limited to technical gestures, but also encompasses a coordination and information relay dimension, which is crucial to the patient's overall care.

Daily observation: being the eyes and ears of the care team

Because of their constant presence with patients, nursing auxiliaries are often the first to observe changes in the patient's state of health. Whether it's the appearance of new symptoms, a worsening of existing clinical signs, or subtle changes in the patient's behavior, these daily observations are essential to management. For example, in a gastroenterology department, the caregiver may notice an increase in abdominal pain, changes in intestinal transit (diarrhea or constipation), signs of dehydration linked to frequent vomiting, or eating difficulties. These observations, which may seem minor at first glance, must be quickly relayed to the nurse and doctor so that they can be integrated into the medical follow-up.

The caregiver's ability to observe and report these elements accurately is therefore crucial. It's not just a question of observing facts, but also of interpreting them in the patient's overall context. For example, a change in stool color or consistency may indicate digestive bleeding or malabsorption, requiring a rapid response. Similarly, signs such as increased fatigue or loss of appetite may signal a more subtle deterioration in health. Thanks to their direct and frequent contact with the patient, caregivers often become the person who alerts the nursing team to clinical decompensation, enabling early intervention.

Communication with the care team: an essential relay role

The transmission of information between the caregiver and other members of the care team is a key element in the coordination of care. Caregivers work in close collaboration with nurses, doctors, and sometimes other professionals such as dieticians or psychologists. They play a relay role, providing valuable information that influences clinical decisions.

One of the most widely used tools for transmitting information is the care record, where the orderly notes down all observations: temperature readings, blood pressure readings, changes in vital parameters, but also more qualitative information such as patient complaints about pain, emotional state, or particular reactions to treatments. This rigorously recorded data enables the entire medical team to monitor the evolution of the patient's state of health in real time.

Oral transmissions, particularly during shift changeovers, are also a key moment for sharing information. At these times, the orderly informs his or her colleagues about changes in the patient's condition, the care already provided, any complications, and any adjustments to be made. This is a crucial moment for ensuring continuity of care without a break in information, especially in situations where teams change frequently, such as during night shifts.

Effective communication also requires the ability to synthesize information. The caregiver must be able to convey the most important elements quickly and clearly, while adapting his or her discourse to the needs of different interlocutors. For example, when communicating with a doctor, the caregiver will focus on observable clinical data (pain, vital parameters), while with nurses, he or she may also include more practical details of care provided or to be provided.

Connecting with patients: an intermediary role

The nursing auxiliary also acts as an intermediary between the patient and the nursing team, facilitating communication between them. Many patients, particularly those suffering from complex or chronic pathologies, have questions, concerns or difficulties understanding certain medical explanations. The caregiver, thanks to his or her close relationship with the patient, often becomes the person to whom the latter confides his or her doubts or misunderstandings. These may be questions about a treatment, the management of side effects, or concerns about the evolution of the disease.

In these situations, the caregiver has a mediating role. He or she must convey the patient's concerns to the medical team, while helping the patient to better understand his or her treatment or to anticipate the next steps. This role is particularly important in situations of emotional vulnerability, when the patient feels helpless in the face of illness, or finds it difficult to express his or her needs directly to the doctors. By relaying this information, the caregiver enables a more human and personalized approach to care, focused on the patient's specific needs and expectations.

Treatment monitoring and adjustments

Another crucial aspect of the caregiver's role in transmitting information concerns the monitoring of ongoing treatments. In a gastroenterology department, patients may be receiving a wide range of treatments, from simple antiemetics to heavier treatments such as infusions of immunosuppressants or biotherapies. Caregivers are often the first to notice the side effects of these treatments, such as allergic reactions, exacerbated digestive disorders, or signs of tolerance or intolerance to the treatment.

By closely monitoring the patient's reactions to treatments, the caregiver plays a decisive role in adjusting therapeutic protocols. If a patient complains of increased nausea after taking a drug, or if signs of extreme fatigue appear after an infusion, the caregiver must quickly inform the nursing and medical team so that an assessment can be made and treatment adjusted if necessary.

- Teamwork with doctors, nurses, physiotherapists and dieticians

Teamwork in the hospital environment, particularly in gastroenterology, is based on close collaboration between various healthcare professionals: doctors, nurses, physiotherapists, dieticians and nursing assistants. Each member of this multi-disciplinary team brings specific and complementary skills to the table, which together ensure comprehensive, personalized and effective patient care. In this context, communication, coordination and mutual trust are key elements in guaranteeing quality care, meeting patients' needs and promoting their recovery.

Working with doctors

As the conductor of medical care, the doctor is responsible for diagnosis, prescribing treatment and overall monitoring of the patient's state of health. However, he or she cannot accomplish this task effectively without constant communication with the other members of the care team, particularly the nursing assistants. The latter play an essential role in feeding back information from their daily observation of patients.

Caregivers are often the first to detect signs of deteriorating health, such as severe abdominal pain, repeated vomiting, changes in bowel habits, or signs of dehydration. These observations are crucial for the doctor, who can adjust treatments or prescribe additional tests. This daily interaction between caregiver and doctor not only ensures responsiveness to changing symptoms, but also guarantees that care is tailored to the specific needs of each patient.

In emergency situations, this collaboration becomes even more essential. For example, in the event of digestive haemorrhage or intestinal obstruction, the caregiver must react quickly, inform the doctor, and assist in the implementation of first aid measures. Thanks to this effective coordination, the team can intervene without delay and limit the risk of serious complications.

A constant link with nurses

The working relationship between orderlies and nurses is particularly close. The nurse, in charge of technical care (administering medication, setting up infusions, monitoring vital parameters), works closely with the orderly to ensure continuity of care. This duo, who share patients' daily lives, form the core of clinical care.

The orderly assists the nurse in a number of tasks, such as preparing the patient for certain treatments, monitoring clinical signs after an operation, or managing medical devices such as nasogastric tubes and catheters. This cooperation ensures an efficient division of responsibilities and comprehensive follow-up, especially when the workload is heavy.

Communication between nurse and caregiver is essential to ensure that all aspects of care are taken into account. For example, when the caregiver notices a worsening of symptoms or the patient reports discomfort, he or she passes this information on to the nurse, who can then adjust treatments or take additional measures. This constant dialogue ensures close, ongoing monitoring of the patient's state of health, helping to prevent complications and improve comfort.

Complementarity with physiotherapists

Physiotherapists often work with hospitalized patients, particularly those suffering from serious digestive pathologies requiring prolonged immobilization. Their role is to prevent complications associated with prolonged bed rest, such as pulmonary infections, venous thrombosis and bedsores, as well as to help patients maintain their mobility and regain their physical autonomy.

In this context, collaboration between the nursing auxiliary and the physiotherapist is essential. The caregiver prepares the patient for rehabilitation sessions, making him/her comfortable and ensuring that he/she is ready for the procedure. They also help to ensure the patient's safety during mobilizations, sometimes accompanying the physiotherapist in his or her movements, particularly for the most fragile or dependent patients.

After the session, the caregiver continues to monitor the patient's condition, paying attention to signs of fatigue or pain, and reporting his or her observations to the physiotherapist or nurse. This post-session follow-up is essential for adapting exercises and ensuring that rehabilitation takes place in the best possible conditions. Thanks to this collaboration, patients benefit from a comprehensive approach that combines medical care, physical rehabilitation and day-to-day support.

Coordination with dieticians

Gastroenterological pathologies often have a direct impact on patient nutrition. Malabsorption, specific diets (residue-free, gluten-free, fiber-low), or the need for enteral or parenteral nutrition are frequent realities in this field. The role of the dietician is therefore crucial in establishing appropriate dietary plans, guaranteeing the necessary nutritional intake and monitoring any deficiencies.

As a local professional, the nursing auxiliary plays a crucial role in implementing dietary recommendations. He/she ensures that the patient complies with dietary instructions, helps with meals if necessary, and observes the patient's reactions to food (nausea, vomiting, pain, intolerances). This information is then passed on to the dietician, who can adjust the nutritional plan according to the caregiver's observations.

In addition, in situations where oral nutrition is difficult or impossible, the caregiver actively participates in the management of enteral nutrition devices, monitoring probes and ensuring they are working properly. They also monitor signs of complications, such as local infections, diarrhea or digestive disorders, and report them to the dieticians and medical team.

The importance of interprofessional communication

In a hospital setting, inter-professional communication is the key to coordinated, effective care. Each healthcare professional, whether doctor, nurse, physiotherapist, dietician or care assistant, brings specific skills to the table, but it is their ability to work together that guarantees comprehensive care tailored to the patient's needs.

The caregiver occupies a central position in this network, as he or she is often the person who spends the most time at the patient's bedside, and has invaluable information on his or her day-to-day state of health. By relaying this information clearly and accurately to all team members, the caregiver helps to ensure effective care coordination. It also ensures that all aspects of the patient's well-being are taken into account, whether in terms of physical condition, nutritional needs, comfort or rehabilitation.

Team meetings and oral and written communications between healthcare professionals are crucial to ensuring fluid communication. During these exchanges, each team member can share his or her observations and recommendations, enabling a coherent care plan to be drawn up, adapted to the patient's evolving state of health.

3 Human and interpersonal skills

• Active listening and empathy with patients who are often anxious or vulnerable

Active listening and empathy are essential qualities in the caregiver-patient relationship, particularly in the field of gastroenterology, where patients are often anxious, vulnerable and confronted with pathologies that can be chronic, incapacitating or serious. These human skills play a fundamental role in patients' well-being, and help to create a climate of trust that is essential to quality care. Active listening and empathy not only help to meet patients' emotional and psychological needs, but also foster more effective communication, essential to fully understanding their symptoms and concerns.

Active listening: more than just a verbal exchange

Active listening means paying full attention to what the patient says, but also to what is left unsaid, to gestures and body language. This involves not only hearing what the patient says, but also understanding the deeper meaning of what he or she is saying, his or her underlying emotions, and needs that are not directly expressed. The caregiver, often on the front line of day-to-day care, plays a crucial role in this listening, as he or she spends the most time with the patient and can pick up on subtle signals.

When dealing with patients suffering from digestive pathologies, active listening is particularly important. These patients, whether suffering from chronic inflammatory bowel disease, digestive cancers, or functional disorders such as irritable bowel syndrome, are often confronted with disabling, unpredictable and sometimes taboo symptoms, such as abdominal pain, frequent diarrhea or vomiting. These symptoms, combined with the uncertainty of the disease's evolution or the constraints associated with treatment, generate anxiety and a feeling of vulnerability. Active listening gives a voice to these concerns, allowing patients to express themselves freely, without judgment, and creating a reassuring space for dialogue.

The caregiver needs to know how to ask the right questions, rephrase what the patient has said to make sure he or she has understood, and show that he or she is attentive to the patient's needs. For example, a patient complaining of abdominal pain may be reluctant to detail the intensity of his symptoms for fear of worrying or being misunderstood. Active listening helps to probe these points, by asking open-ended questions such as: "Can you explain to me at what time of day these pains occur?" or "How do you feel these pains? Is it discomfort or intense pain? This approach helps the patient to feel listened to and understood, while providing the care team with valuable information for adjusting care.

Empathy: putting yourself in the patient's shoes

Empathy, on the other hand, is the ability to put oneself in the patient's shoes, to understand how they feel, not only physically, but also emotionally. This is a particularly crucial quality in gastroenterology, where patients can feel particularly vulnerable due to the intimate nature of their symptoms. Digestive disorders, often associated with bodily functions such as digestion, elimination or feeding, can generate great embarrassment or shame in patients, especially in a hospital setting where their privacy is often reduced.

Empathy means recognizing these emotions and responding appropriately. For example, a patient suffering from chronic diarrhoea may be embarrassed to ask for help in changing his or her sheets or cleaning up. An empathetic response involves approaching the situation in a caring, non-judgmental way, explaining to the patient that these situations are normal in the context of his or her pathology, and that there's no need to feel embarrassed. The caregiver may say something like, "I understand that this can be difficult, but please know that we're here to help you and that it's part of our job to ensure your comfort and well-being." This approach reduces the patient's anxiety and strengthens the relationship of trust.

Empathy also means recognizing the emotional impact of chronic or serious digestive diseases. Patients suffering from digestive cancers or illnesses such as Crohn's disease may be faced with heavy treatment, repeated surgery, or periods of uncertainty about their prognosis. These patients often experience moments of discouragement, fear or even anger. The caregiver, by showing empathy, can offer invaluable support, recognizing the difficulty of these situations and offering a sympathetic ear. It's not just a matter of providing technical care, but also a human presence, capable of understanding the patient's emotions and accompanying them through these difficult moments.

Creating an environment of trust

Active listening and empathy are also the foundations of a trusting environment, where patients feel comfortable expressing their needs, fears and expectations. When patients feel that their concerns are taken into account and their emotions respected, they are more inclined to communicate openly with the healthcare team, to express their symptoms more accurately and to participate actively in their own treatment.

An anxious patient, for example, may be reluctant to report treatment side-effects or changes in symptoms for fear of disturbing others. By creating a climate of trust, the caregiver enables the patient to understand that every piece of information is important for his or her follow-up, and that his or her feelings are legitimate. A patient who feels listened to and understood will be more inclined to cooperate, to ask questions about his or her treatment, and to follow medical recommendations with greater serenity.

This environment of trust is particularly important for patients at the end of life, or those with serious illnesses, who may have specific emotional needs. Empathy is essential to accompany these patients on their care journey, respecting their wishes, limitations and fears. Active listening enables us to pick up signals about their emotional state, how they feel about pain, or their anxiety about the future, so that we can adapt our care and offer them appropriate emotional support.

Strengthening the caregiver-patient bond

Active listening and empathy also strengthen the bond between caregiver and patient, making care more personalized and humane. By showing patients that they are taken into account in their entirety, beyond their physical symptoms, the caregiver participates in a holistic approach to care. This bond of trust promotes not only the patient's well-being, but also his or her recovery, as an emotionally and psychologically supported patient often responds better to treatment and demonstrates greater resilience in the face of illness.

The caregiver's daily proximity to the patient often makes him or her the first point of contact. It is in this direct relationship that bonds of trust and empathy are forged. When the caregiver takes the time to listen, understand and respond to the patient's needs with sensitivity, he or she becomes an essential support, both practically and psychologically.

- Stress and emergency management

Managing stress and emergency situations is an integral part of the skills required in the hospital environment, particularly in specialties such as gastroenterology, where patients can be confronted with sudden and potentially serious complications. Emergencies can occur at any time: digestive haemorrhages, intestinal occlusions, perforations or decompensations of chronic diseases. Effective response to these situations depends not only on the speed of medical intervention, but also on the ability of the care team to maintain composure, organize care and manage the stress associated with these critical moments.

Understanding and anticipating emergency situations

In gastroenterology, emergency situations are varied and sometimes unexpected. Certain pathologies, such as acute digestive haemorrhage or severe pancreatitis, can degenerate rapidly and put the patient's life at risk. An essential part of emergency management is anticipating and recognizing the warning signs. For example, a sudden drop in blood pressure, the appearance of bloody vomit (hematemesis), black stools (melena) or severe abdominal pain may be the first signs of a serious complication requiring immediate attention.

The nursing auxiliary, on the front line of patient monitoring, plays a key role in this surveillance. By being alert to subtle changes in the patient's state of health, they can quickly alert the medical team. This involves recognizing the clinical signs of concern and understanding their significance, even if it is not his or her role to make a diagnosis. Effective emergency management therefore depends on the ability to identify these signs quickly and react without delay.

Reactivity and organization in emergency situations

When emergencies arise, the speed and organization of the response are crucial. Each member of the care team has a well-defined role, and coordination is essential to ensure effective care. Faced with a digestive hemorrhage, for example, the caregiver may be responsible for preparing the patient for an emergency endoscopy, checking vital signs continuously, or ensuring that the necessary equipment, such as catheters or infusions, is available and ready to use.

In these moments of crisis, stress management is paramount. It's easy to become overwhelmed by the intensity of the situation, but the caregiver must remain calm to ensure precise actions and effective communication with the rest of the team. Good preparation and clear organization help reduce stress. This includes knowledge of emergency protocols, mastery of medical equipment, and familiarity with resuscitation or blood transfusion procedures.

One of the key aspects of stress management in emergency situations is the ability to focus on immediate priorities. It is important not to lose focus in the face of an emergency, but to stay focused on the actions needed in the short term, such as stabilizing the patient's vital parameters, managing pain, or preparing equipment for rapid intervention. The ability to prioritize actions is essential to avoid wasting time in the crucial first minutes of an emergency.

Clear, effective communication

In any emergency situation, clear and rapid communication is essential to ensure consistent and coordinated care. Caregivers must be able to convey important information concisely and accurately. This means knowing how to report worrying signs immediately, answering doctors' and nurses' questions, and following instructions precisely.

Good communication also helps avoid misunderstandings or errors, which can be costly in terms of time and safety for the patient. The caregiver must ensure that essential information - such as the patient's history, recent symptoms, or current treatments - is shared with the entire care team. In moments of intense stress, it's also important to take the time to rephrase instructions if necessary, to make sure they've been properly understood.

Communication with the patient, even in an emergency situation, is also crucial. Although emergencies call for swift action, it's essential to bear in mind that the patient may be feeling extremely vulnerable and anxious. Taking the time to briefly explain what's happening, even in just a few words, and reassuring the patient that he or she is in good hands, can considerably reduce stress and facilitate care. A phrase as simple as "We'll take care of you, we'll manage the situation" can have a calming effect in a context where the patient feels distraught.

Personal stress management in emergency situations

Managing personal stress is a key issue for healthcare professionals, as it is essential to remain effective even under pressure. Stress, if not properly managed, can impair concentration, lead to errors and increase the risk of burnout. To avoid this, several strategies can be adopted by the caregiver and the rest of the care team.

First and foremost, regular training in emergency situations enables them to better anticipate and manage stress when a real emergency arises. By regularly practicing emergency scenarios, caregivers develop reflexes that enable them to react with confidence and efficiency. What's more, in-depth knowledge of protocols and equipment boosts self-confidence and reduces anxiety.

Secondly, it's important to take a step back after an emergency situation to analyze what went well and what could be improved. This allows you to learn from each experience and prepare even better for the future. What's more, sharing your feelings with colleagues after an emergency helps to defuse some of the accumulated stress and strengthen team cohesion. It also helps avoid the emotional overload that can result from managing repeated crises.

Finally, daily stress management techniques, such as controlled breathing, mindfulness, or the organization of rest periods, are essential for maintaining emotional balance and preventing exhaustion. Taking care of yourself, physically and mentally, is essential if you are to respond effectively to emergencies.

Preventing emergencies through increased surveillance

One of the best ways to manage emergencies is to prevent them as much as possible. Careful monitoring of vital signs, attention to patient complaints, and ongoing communication with the medical team can detect early warning signs before a situation becomes critical. For example, in the event of persistent diarrhea or frequent vomiting, the caregiver can alert the team to an increased risk of dehydration or electrolyte imbalance, enabling them to intervene before decompensation occurs.

Prevention also involves patient education. The caregiver, in collaboration with the rest of the team, can explain to the patient the warning signs to watch out for and the measures to take to avoid a worsening of his or her condition. Keeping patients well-informed about their illness, their treatments and the precautions to be taken at home can often prevent avoidable emergencies.

4 Ethics and confidentiality: essential principles

• Respect for patient dignity and privacy

Respect for patient dignity and privacy is a fundamental principle of all healthcare practice, particularly in the field of gastroenterology, where care often involves situations of extreme vulnerability. Patients confronted with illnesses that affect intimate aspects of their bodies, such as digestion or elimination, may feel embarrassed or even ashamed by the examinations or treatments they undergo. In this context, preserving patients' dignity and privacy is not only an ethical requirement, but also a key factor in their psychological well-being and the quality of their care.

Patient dignity: a fundamental right

Dignity is an intrinsic right of every individual, regardless of their state of health. As caregivers, respecting this dignity means considering each patient as a whole person, with his or her own values, needs and expectations, and not simply as a "medical case". This means recognizing their humanity, taking into account their emotions and fears, and treating them with respect and kindness.

In gastroenterological care, patients can feel particularly vulnerable, as symptoms and treatments touch on bodily functions that are often taboo. For example, a colonoscopy or endoscopy, although routine for caregivers, may be perceived by patients as an intrusion into their privacy. Similarly, digestive disorders such as diarrhoea, vomiting or incontinence can cause great embarrassment, and even a feeling of worthlessness. In such situations, it is essential to show patients that they are being treated with respect, by explaining each stage of care and maintaining a framework of dignity.

Respecting patients' dignity also means listening to them. Letting patients express their fears, questions or reservations about certain treatments not only reassures them, but also recognizes them as active participants in their own care. For example, when a patient expresses concerns about undergoing a procedure such as gastroscopy, it's important to take the time to answer their questions, reassure them about the procedure, and respect their pace, while explaining the benefits of the care.

Preserving privacy in care

Physical intimacy is a crucial aspect of respect for the individual, particularly during care involving examinations or procedures affecting sensitive areas of the body. In gastroenterology, many medical procedures require examination of the abdominal, rectal or anal regions, and can create a feeling of vulnerability in the patient. Preserving this intimacy, even in medical situations where the body is widely exposed, is essential to maintaining respect and trust.

It is therefore essential to adopt a delicate and respectful approach, taking care to explain each procedure before carrying it out, and systematically seeking the patient's consent before any intervention. For example, before performing a colonoscopy or nasogastric tube insertion, it is essential to inform the patient of the procedure and assure him or her that every precaution will be taken to minimize discomfort and respect his or her privacy.

Respect for privacy also includes simple but essential gestures, such as ensuring that sheets are used to cover parts of the body not involved in the examination, closing the bedroom door or drawing a curtain during care, and avoiding untimely interruptions. These little gestures help patients to feel protected, even in situations where they have to be undressed or exposed for medical reasons.

Emotional intimacy: a dimension not to be neglected

In addition to physical privacy, it's important to preserve the patient's emotional intimacy. This is achieved by the way caregivers handle personal or medical information. Patients need to feel that their care is treated with discretion, and that their medical information is shared only with the professionals directly involved in their care.

At times when the patient expresses emotions, such as anxiety or fear, the caregiver must know how to respond with empathy and kindness, without judging or minimizing his or her feelings. Emotional intimacy also concerns the way in which discussions about the patient's health are conducted: they should be done in private, in a setting conducive to confidentiality, and not in a public place or in front of other patients. This reinforces the patient's sense of trust in the healthcare team.

For example, a patient suffering from a chronic illness such as Crohn's disease may have fears about his future, the evolution of his pathology, or the impact of the disease on his daily life. Allowing such patients to express themselves freely, while respecting their confidentiality, helps to preserve their emotional intimacy and support them in this vulnerable phase.

Creating a climate of trust

Respecting patients' dignity and privacy is also a way of strengthening the relationship of trust between caregiver and patient. When patients feel that their bodies, emotions and personal information are respected, they are more likely to cooperate fully in their care and accept the treatment offered. This trust is particularly important in situations where treatments may be invasive or uncomfortable.

Trust also depends on transparency and communication. By clearly explaining to the patient the reasons for the procedure, the expected benefits, and any associated discomforts, the caregiver enables the patient to feel involved and informed, thus reinforcing his or her cooperation. For example, when preparing for a colonoscopy, a precise explanation of the steps to be followed, the effects of laxative treatment and the course of the examination helps to reassure patients and reduce their apprehension.

Respecting patient choice

Respecting patients' dignity also means recognizing their right to participate actively in decisions concerning their health. Patients have the right to express their preferences, refusals or doubts about certain treatments or interventions. This dimension of autonomy is fundamental, as it places the patient at the center of his or her care, as the principal actor.

In certain situations, a patient may choose to refuse an examination or treatment, even if it is deemed necessary by the medical team. The role of the caregiver is to respect this choice, while providing the information necessary for the patient to make an informed decision. This respect for patients' autonomy and choices enhances their dignity, by recognizing their right to decide for themselves.

- Personal and medical data management

Managing patients' personal and medical data is a fundamental aspect of healthcare practice, involving both ethical and legal responsibilities. In a medical context such as that of gastroenterology, where the information collected can be particularly sensitive, the protection of such data is of paramount importance. Confidentiality, respect for privacy and the security of information are principles that guarantee patients' trust in the healthcare team. Good data management means both respecting patients' rights and ensuring high-quality medical care, where access to information is both secure and limited to those concerned.

The importance of confidentiality

The confidentiality of personal and medical data is a fundamental right of patients, enshrined in numerous international and national legislations, such as the General Data Protection Regulation

(GDPR) in Europe. This right to confidentiality applies to all information relating to the patient's state of health, but also to their personal data, such as their identity, address, or contact details. In gastroenterology, where diseases affect intimate aspects of the body, such as digestive functions, discreet management of this data is essential to respect the patient's dignity and protect his or her privacy.

Patients need to be assured that the information they share with their medical team, whether it relates to their symptoms, personal history, or treatments, will only be used in the context of their care. Data management must therefore be rigorous, with clear protocols to prevent unauthorized access. This includes not only the protection of paper medical records, but also the security of computer databases, where medical information is stored. Any leakage or mismanagement of this data can have serious consequences, not only for the institution's reputation, but above all for patient privacy.

Data access: who is concerned?

In the context of medical care, only those people directly involved in the patient's treatment should have access to his or her personal and medical data. This includes doctors, nurses, care assistants and, in some cases, other healthcare professionals such as physiotherapists or dieticians, depending on the patient's specific needs. This principle of limited access ensures that confidential information is not disclosed to third parties not involved in the treatment.

In daily practice, the nursing auxiliary plays a key role in managing the information transmitted between the patient and the medical team. They are in the front line when it comes to observing changes in the patient's condition, gathering information on symptoms or feelings, and passing it on to the team. However, this transmission of information must always respect confidentiality. For example, an orderly cannot discuss the details of a patient's illness outside the care areas or with people outside the care team.

Confidentiality also includes protection from prying eyes within the hospital itself. When discussing a patient's state of health, whether in a team meeting or during transmissions between caregivers, it is important to ensure that these exchanges take place in a private environment. Discussing a patient's state of health in a corridor, in the presence of other patients or visitors, contravenes the rules of confidentiality and can affect the relationship of trust between the patient and his or her care team.

Electronic and paper medical records management

In modern hospitals, the management of medical data is often based on the use of electronic records. These systems enable fast, efficient access to patient medical information, while reducing the risk of paper documents being lost or damaged. However, this digitization of records requires strict security measures to protect sensitive data.

IT systems for managing medical records must be secured by protective protocols, such as the use of strong passwords, limited access according to the responsibilities of each caregiver, and data encryption systems. Healthcare professionals, including caregivers, must be trained to use these tools responsibly and securely. For example, it is essential that each user logs out of the computer system after accessing a patient's data, to prevent unauthorized access by others.

As far as paper files are concerned, although increasingly dematerialized, they are still present in certain departments. Their management must also be strictly controlled. Files must be stored in secure cabinets, accessible only to authorized personnel. They must never be left in view of unauthorized persons, such as visitors or other patients, and must be regularly updated and archived in compliance with current regulations.

Medical data transmission: precision and discretion

The transmission of medical data, whether oral or written, is a key moment in the management of patient information. As the intermediary between the patient and the nursing team, orderlies must be precise and meticulous when transmitting information. Whether reporting symptoms observed, treatments administered or patient complaints, the data transmitted must be accurate and reported in a professional manner.

Oral transmissions, often carried out during team changes, must take place in a confidential setting, away from prying eyes and ears. What's more, they must be concise and to the point, to ensure continuity of care without divulging information that is superfluous or irrelevant to immediate care.

In the case of written transmission, such as observation reports or file updates, confidentiality remains a key principle. Notes recorded in files must be accurate and factual, without personal judgment or inappropriate comments. Rigorous documentation ensures the traceability of care and facilitates coordination between the various parties involved, while respecting the confidentiality of patient data.

Patient consent and data management

Respecting patient consent is another fundamental pillar of personal and medical data management. Patients must be informed of how their data is collected, used and shared, and must give their explicit consent to any use of their data outside the strictly medical context. This includes, for example, participation in clinical studies or the transmission of their information to other medical institutions.

Patients also have the right to know who can access their data, and for what purpose. For example, in the context of a specialized consultation, the attending physician may need to pass on certain medical information to a gastroenterologist or surgeon. However, this sharing must always be done with the informed consent of the patient, who must be informed of the purpose of this transmission.

Data protection after processing

Data management doesn't stop at the end of medical treatment. Patients' medical information must be kept securely, even after they have been discharged from hospital or their treatment has been completed. Regulations vary from country to country, but in general, medical records must be kept for a specified period, and then archived or securely destroyed once this period has elapsed.

Compliance with these rules ensures that personal data does not fall into the wrong hands, even many years after the end of care. Healthcare institutions are responsible for the proper management of these archives, and must put in place clear protocols to ensure that records are properly protected, whether digital or physical.

Chapter 3

Daily management of gastroenterology patients

1 Welcoming a patient to the gastroenterology department

- Welcoming the patient: initial approach and building confidence

Welcoming the patient is a crucial stage in the care process, as it constitutes the first approach and marks the beginning of the relationship between the patient and the care team. It is at this point that first impressions are made, and that trust - a central element of quality care - begins to be established. In gastroenterology, where patients are often confronted with illnesses that touch on intimate and potentially embarrassing aspects of their health, the way in which they are greeted plays an essential role in reassuring them, putting them at ease, and preparing them to accept care under the best possible conditions.

The first approach: creating a climate of empathy and listening

Welcoming patients begins as soon as they arrive at the hospital or doctor's surgery. The first approach is crucial in establishing a climate of trust and security. Patients, often stressed or worried about their illness or the examination they are about to undergo, need to be treated with kindness and attention. From the outset, the attitude of the health-care team, and in particular the nursing auxiliary, must be one of empathy and listening.

It's essential to greet the patient with a smile, a reassuring tone, and gestures that show you're there to support them. This benevolent approach quickly dissipates some of the stress the patient may be feeling. For example, a simple "Hello, my name is [first name], I'll be looking after you today. How are you feeling?" can be enough to establish a human connection and show the patient that he or she is not just a "case" or a number, but a person whose needs and emotions are taken into account.

From this first approach, it's also important to create a space for listening. Patients, particularly in gastroenterology, may have concerns about their state of health, fears about invasive examinations such as colonoscopy, or questions about their treatment. Caregivers need to listen carefully, pay attention to non-verbal cues, and be available to answer initial questions or reassure patients about the next stage in their care.

Inform to reassure

Information plays a vital role in building patient confidence. A patient who is well-informed about the course of treatment or examinations he or she is about to undergo will be more serene and more likely to cooperate. The welcome is therefore an opportunity to provide clear explanations adapted to the patient's level of understanding. In gastroenterology, examinations can often be perceived as invasive or intimidating, whether it's an endoscopy, a colonoscopy, or the insertion of a nasogastric tube.

It's important to explain to the patient, step by step, what's going to happen. For example, in the case of a colonoscopy, you might explain: "You'll be seated comfortably on your side. The examination may be a little uncomfortable, but it won't be painful. We'll be here to support you throughout the procedure, and if you feel the slightest discomfort, please don't hesitate to let us know." This type of explanation helps reduce patient anxiety by giving them greater control over the situation.

The use of simple, non-medical terms, while respecting the patient's intelligence and dignity, is essential to avoid losing him or her in overly technical explanations. It is also useful to check that the patient has understood what has been explained, by asking open-ended questions such as: "Do you have any questions about what is going to happen?

Respecting the patient's rhythm

Every patient is different, and some may need more time to adapt to their medical environment. Reception is the time to respect this rhythm, without rushing things. A patient who feels hurried or rushed can quickly lose confidence and become reluctant to collaborate. For example, if a patient seems particularly anxious about undergoing an examination, the orderly can offer to give them a few extra minutes to relax, discuss their apprehensions, or even explain the diagnostic benefits of the examination.

This respect for rhythm is particularly important with the elderly or patients suffering from chronic pathologies, who may feel tired or emotionally vulnerable. Giving them time, not forcing them to move too quickly through the care process, and being patient with their questions or hesitations is a mark of respect and consideration that helps establish a lasting relationship of trust.

Creating an environment conducive to confidentiality and privacy

When welcoming patients, it is also crucial to ensure that their confidentiality and privacy are preserved. Entering the hospital or consultation can be a time when the patient feels exposed, especially if he or she is asked to talk about symptoms or medical history in a space where others can hear. The caregiver must ensure that these discussions take place in a discreet environment, away from prying eyes or ears.

In the case of a hospitalized patient, the reception in the room must be carried out in such a way as to guarantee his or her privacy. Closing the door or drawing the curtains when the patient is first admitted, explaining that he or she can ask for a moment's peace and quiet, or informing him or her of the times when he or she will be called upon for treatment are all gestures that help to preserve this privacy. This also helps to reduce stress and reinforce the patient's sense of security.

Humanizing care

Finally, the welcome is an opportunity to humanize the caregiver-patient relationship, by showing the patient that, despite the sometimes intimidating medical context, he or she is first and foremost a person with emotions, expectations and specific needs. This humanization is achieved through small gestures of consideration, such as the use of the patient's first name, warm eye contact, or simple gestures like adjusting a pillow or offering water.

By being attentive to these details, the caregiver helps to humanize the patient's experience, making him or her feel less depersonalized in a care system that is sometimes perceived as impersonal. This attention to the individual, beyond the sick body, creates a strong, lasting bond between patient and healthcare team. For example, asking the patient if he or she slept well the night before, or if there is anything he or she needs before the examination begins, shows that we take into account the patient's comfort and well-being as a whole.

- Patient room set-up: comfort and safety

Room placement is a key stage in a patient's hospitalization, and goes beyond simply allocating a bed. It is essential to ensure the patient's physical comfort and safety, as well as to provide an environment conducive to recovery. In a gastroenterology department, where patients may be confronted with uncomfortable symptoms and heavy treatments, this settling-in phase must be handled with care and humanity. The aim is not only to ensure that the patient feels at ease, but also to put in place all safety measures to prevent risks associated with their illness or state of weakness.

Welcoming patients to their rooms: the first step to well-being

The process of settling into the patient's room begins as soon as the patient enters the room, which will be his or her living space during the hospital stay. For patients, who may be anxious about their illness or hospitalization, this moment must be an opportunity to reassure them and offer them a warm, reassuring care environment. The nursing auxiliary plays a central role here, welcoming the patient in a friendly manner and explaining how his or her stay in the room will unfold.

The first step is to accompany the patient to bed, helping them to settle in if necessary, especially if they have mobility difficulties. This support is crucial for patients suffering from abdominal pain, exhaustion due to their illness or ongoing treatment, or for those who are elderly or in a weakened condition. The caregiver must ensure that the patient is comfortably installed in a position that minimizes discomfort, for example by adjusting the height of the bed or placing pillows to support certain parts of the body.

The caregiver must also explain to the patient how the room's equipment works, such as the medical bed, call devices to alert staff in case of need, or light or air-conditioning settings. This information is essential to enable the patient to feel in control of his or her environment, reducing anxiety and increasing feelings of security.

Patient comfort: physical and psychological well-being

Patient comfort is a top priority during room set-up, as it contributes directly to their well-being and recovery. In gastroenterology, many patients suffer from symptoms such as abdominal pain, nausea, bloating or diarrhea, which can make hospitalization particularly difficult. To help them cope with these discomforts, it's essential to offer them a care environment conducive to rest and relaxation.

Bed positioning is a key factor in this quest for comfort. The caregiver must adjust the bed to relieve muscular tension and prevent pain. This may include raising the head of the bed to facilitate breathing, or to limit gastro-oesophageal reflux, which is common in patients with digestive disorders. Pillows and blankets should also be arranged to support sensitive areas, especially in patients confined to bed for long periods.

Comfort also involves room temperature, lighting and noise levels. The caregiver can ask the patient if he or she would like to adjust the temperature or brightness to create a soothing environment. It is also important to ensure that the room remains a quiet place, free from excessive noise that could disturb the patient's sleep or rest.

Finally, to enhance the patient's psychological well-being, the caregiver may suggest personalizing the room by bringing in personal objects, such as books, photos or an electronic device, to make it more familiar and less cold. These little touches help create a bond between the patient and the nursing team, reinforcing the relationship of trust and humanity that is essential throughout the stay.

Patient safety: preventing hospital-related risks

In addition to comfort, patient safety is another major priority when it comes to room set-up. Hospitalized patients, particularly those suffering from gastroenterological illnesses, can be fragile and prone to complications such as falls, bedsores and treatment side-effects. It is therefore essential to take all necessary measures to prevent these risks from the moment they arrive in their room.

One of the first things to do is to ensure that the patient has call devices at hand to alert staff in case of need. The caregiver must explain to the patient how to use this equipment and check that it is functional. This simple but essential gesture ensures that the patient can call for help at any time, particularly if he or she feels unwell, needs to get up to go to the toilet, or experiences sudden pain.

Preventing falls is another important safety issue, especially for elderly, weak or sedated patients. The caregiver must ensure that the bed is set at a safe height, that side rails are in place if necessary, and that the room is clear of any obstacles that could impede the patient's movements, such as electrical wires or objects on the floor. It is also advisable to check that the patient has non-slip footwear to avoid any risk of slipping when moving around.

For patients on long-term bed rest, pressure sore prevention is an essential aspect of safety. The caregiver must ensure that the mattress is suitable and, if necessary, that special equipment such as an anti-decubitus mattress is available. Regular mobilization of the patient must also be planned, in collaboration with the nursing team, to avoid prolonged pressure points.

Adapting the environment to the patient's specific needs

Each patient has specific needs depending on his or her pathology, state of health and mobility. When setting up in the room, the caregiver must therefore adapt the environment to these particularities. For example, a patient suffering from a chronic inflammatory bowel disease, such as Crohn's, may need rapid access to the toilet. In such cases, it is crucial to ensure that the room is close to a bathroom, or to install an auxiliary device such as a bedpan or commode near the bed.

In addition, some patients require special medical devices, such as infusions, enteral nutrition pumps or nasogastric tubes. In such cases, the caregiver must ensure that these devices are installed in the best possible way, so as not to impede the patient's movements, while at the same time guaranteeing that they function properly. Regular monitoring of these devices is also part of the safety measures to be observed.

Inform and reassure patients about their stay

Settling patients into their rooms is also the time to inform them about their stay and the care they will receive. By explaining how the day at the hospital will unfold, and the schedule for meals, medical visits and examinations, the nursing assistant helps to reduce anxiety. Knowing the steps involved in hospitalization helps patients feel more confident and better prepared for what lies ahead.

In addition, this information phase clarifies to the patient that he or she can ask questions at any time, request further explanations, or report any discomfort. Establishing this open communication from the moment the patient settles into the room is essential if they are to feel safe and well cared for.

2 Hygiene and comfort care specific to gastroenterology patients

• Management of colostomies and other ostomies

The management of colostomies and other ostomies is an essential aspect of caregivers' work, particularly in specialties such as gastroenterology, where these procedures are frequent. Stomas, whether colostomies, ileostomies or urostomies, are surgical openings created to allow the evacuation of stool or urine when part of the digestive or urinary system can no longer function normally. Although these operations are often vital, they represent a major upheaval in patients' lives, both physically and psychologically. Accompanying patients with an ostomy requires not only technical skills, but also great empathy and a humanistic approach, as adapting to this new reality is often difficult.

Understanding colostomy and other ostomies

A colostomy is a digestive stoma made in the colon, where part of the intestine is shunted to an opening created in the abdomen to allow evacuation of stool into a collecting pouch. This procedure is indicated in a number of cases, including colorectal cancer, inflammatory bowel diseases such as Crohn's disease or ulcerative colitis, or following trauma or bowel obstruction. Depending on the location of the stoma on the colon, stool consistency varies, from liquid to more solid.

Ileostomies, on the other hand, involve shunting the small intestine into the abdomen, producing a more liquid stool. They are often performed for conditions such as ulcerative colitis, when the entire colon has to be removed. Urostomies, on the other hand, concern the urinary system and are used to drain urine directly from the kidneys to the outside in the event of a problem with the bladder or urinary tract.

In all these cases, ostomies impose a radical change on patients. Not only do they have to get used to living with an ostomy pouch, they also have to learn how to manage this new situation on a daily basis. This is where the role of caregivers becomes crucial, offering technical, educational and psychological support.

Technical aspects of stoma management

From a technical point of view, the management of colostomies and other ostomies involves a number of precise, regular gestures to ensure that the stoma functions properly, prevents complications and maintains hygiene. As soon as the stoma is created, the caregiver and nurse must be trained to take charge of daily care and support the patient in learning how to manage his or her stoma.

One of the first essential steps is to monitor the stoma itself. The opening in the abdomen, called a stoma or "mouth" in Latin, must be regularly inspected to ensure that it is healing properly after surgery. The caregiver must ensure that the color of the stoma is normal (usually pink or bright red, a sign of good blood circulation), that there is no excessive bleeding or signs of infection, and that the size of the stoma remains stable.

Care of the skin around the stoma, called the peristomy, is also a priority. The skin is exposed to stool or urine, which can lead to irritation, infection or ulceration if not properly protected. The caregiver must therefore use suitable products to clean the area and apply skin protection before fitting the ostomy pouch. Collection devices (pouches) must be changed regularly, following a rigorous hygiene protocol to prevent leakage or infection. The tightness of the collection system must be checked at each change to ensure patient comfort and limit unpleasant odors.

Patient learning and empowerment

One of the most important aspects of caring for ostomy patients is education. The aim is to make patients autonomous in the day-to-day management of their stoma, so that they can resume as normal a life as possible. This includes the ability to change the ostomy pouch, to clean the peristomal area correctly, and to recognize the signs of complications.

This learning process can be difficult for the patient, especially in the first few weeks after surgery, when he or she must not only get used to a new body, but also deal with the emotions associated with this transformation. The caregiver plays a fundamental role here, accompanying the patient step by step through this learning process. Patience, pedagogy and encouragement are essential. Demonstrating gestures by calmly explaining each step, and then accompanying the patient as he or she begins to perform the care himself or herself, helps to build confidence.

Training should not be limited to technical gestures. It also includes advice on diet, as certain foods can cause gas, diarrhea or constipation, which can make stoma management more difficult. For example, patients with a colostomy need to be informed about foods that can modulate stool consistency or produce gas, so that they can adapt their diet accordingly.

Taking psychological aspects into account

Beyond the technical aspects, ostomy care must also take into account the psychological dimension. Ostomy patients can experience profound emotional upheaval, ranging from fear and sadness to shame and low self-esteem. Body image is often affected, and some patients may feel "diminutive", or even "different", which can lead to a drop in self-esteem, depressive disorders, or difficulties in social and intimate life.

The role of the caregiver is to support the patient during this adaptation phase, by offering a listening ear and responding to any concerns. Empathy is essential, as every patient reacts differently to a stoma. It's important to normalize the situation by explaining that the stoma is a medical solution that enables people to live better, and sometimes saves lives. Encouraging patients to express their emotions, fears and questions can help defuse certain fears and help them gradually accept this new reality.

In addition, caregivers can refer patients to support groups or ostomy associations, where they can talk to other people living with an ostomy. These groups are often a valuable source of moral support, and help patients realize that they are not alone in this situation.

Preventing and managing complications

Finally, ostomy management includes the prevention and management of complications. Possible complications include skin irritation around the stoma, peristomal infections, hernias or stomal prolapse (when the intestine protrudes excessively through the stoma). Caregivers and nurses must be particularly alert to these complications, and trained to react accordingly.

For example, in the event of skin irritation, it is essential to adapt skin care, use specific protective products, and possibly change the type of pouch used. If infection is suspected, additional samples or medical consultations may be necessary to assess the situation.

- Nasogastric tube management and percutaneous care (PEG)

The management of nasogastric tubes and percutaneous care (PEG, percutaneous endoscopic gastrostomy) is an essential aspect of gastroenterology care, particularly for patients who are unable to obtain adequate oral nutrition. These devices deliver nutrition, hydration and medication directly into the stomach or intestine. Their management requires rigorous technical expertise, as well as particular attention to hygiene and patient comfort. What's more, these procedures can be a source of discomfort or anxiety for patients, requiring an empathetic and reassuring approach on the part of caregivers.

Understanding the nasogastric tube: a temporary but delicate solution

The nasogastric tube (NGT) is a device inserted through the nose into the stomach to enable the administration of nutrients, medication or stomach decompression in the event of frequent vomiting or intestinal obstruction. Although often used as a temporary solution, the nasogastric tube can be uncomfortable for patients, due to the sensation of nasal, pharyngeal and esophageal irritation it causes.

Installing an SNG requires great delicacy and technical skill, as it must be inserted correctly to avoid complications such as aspiration into the airway. The orderly, in collaboration with the nurse, is often responsible for monitoring the catheter once it has been inserted. He or she must ensure that the probe is securely attached and does not cause excessive irritation to the nostrils or throat. It is also important to regularly check the position of the probe to ensure that it has not moved and is still correctly positioned in the stomach.

An essential task is to monitor any complications associated with NGLS, such as infections, nasal irritation or minor bleeding. Checking that the catheter is well tolerated by the patient is essential, particularly by assessing whether he or she shows signs of respiratory distress, nausea or excessive discomfort. If the tube is used to drain gastric contents, it is also crucial to ensure that the tube is aspirated, avoiding any obstruction.

Nasogastric tube care and prevention of complications

Day-to-day management of the nasogastric tube involves a number of steps designed to ensure that it functions properly, while minimizing the risk of infection or irritation. Hygiene is a key element in this process. The caregiver must ensure that the probe insertion area is clean, by regularly cleaning the nostrils and ensuring that the adhesive attachment is replaced if it becomes detached or uncomfortable.

It is also essential to prevent the risk of pulmonary aspiration, which can occur if the tube is displaced or if gastric contents are poorly managed. To this end, the patient should be placed in a semi-seated or seated position during meals or the administration of medication via the tube. This helps to promote the descent of food and liquids into the stomach, while minimizing the risk of reflux or passage into the respiratory tract.

In some cases, the nasogastric tube is used for enteral nutrition, i.e. the administration of liquid nutrients directly into the stomach. The caregiver must ensure that nutrient solutions are administered according to a precise protocol, controlling the flow rate and checking that the patient's tolerance is good. Any symptoms of abdominal distension, nausea or vomiting should be reported immediately, as they may indicate poor digestion of nutrients or a problem with the tube itself.

Percutaneous care management (PCM): a long-term alternative

Percutaneous endoscopic gastrostomy (PEG) is a long-term nutrition device for patients who can no longer sustain oral nutrition due to neurodegenerative diseases, advanced cancers or esophageal obstructions. The gastrostomy tube is inserted directly into the stomach through the abdominal wall, offering a more comfortable and stable solution for patients than the nasogastric tube.

Managing a PEG requires rigorous attention to prevent complications, including infections at the insertion site, gastric leakage or granuloma formation around the opening. Daily care of the PEG site is crucial. The caregiver, in collaboration with the nurse, must carefully clean the area around the probe with antiseptic solutions, and ensure that the skin remains dry and clean. It is also necessary to watch for the appearance of redness, swelling or purulent secretions, possible signs of infection.

The management of nutrition via a PEG must follow strict protocols to ensure that nutrients are administered optimally. Nutrient solutions must be infused at a rate adapted to the patient's needs, while ensuring that the patient is in a semi-seated position during and after administration to avoid reflux. Caregivers should monitor the patient's tolerance, in particular the absence of nausea, abdominal pain or diarrhea, which may indicate poor adaptation to the nutrients or the rate of administration.

Educating patients and their families: a central element of care

Whether using a nasogastric tube or a PEG, one of the key aspects of management is educating the patient and his or her family. While the nasogastric tube is generally temporary, the PEG is often used on a long-term basis, which means that patients or their caregivers must learn to manage the device themselves at home.

The caregiver plays an essential role in this learning phase. The caregiver's role is to explain daily procedures, such as cleaning the insertion site, changing nutrition bags, and monitoring for warning signs. It is important to demonstrate these gestures in the presence of the patient or his or her family, and then to support them in their learning process until they feel confident enough to perform them independently.

Listening and availability are essential elements in this process. Patients and their families may feel at a loss when faced with these medical devices, and the role of caregivers is to reassure them, answer their questions, and offer practical advice to ensure that the management of the catheter or PEG goes smoothly at home.

Taking psychological aspects into account

The presence of a nasogastric tube or PEG can be emotionally difficult to accept. For some patients, these devices can be perceived as a loss of autonomy, or even an attack on their dignity, especially when they have to live with them over a long period of time. It is essential that caregivers are attentive to this psychological dimension, listening to any concerns or feelings of frustration that patients may express.

Empathy and benevolence are essential attitudes when accompanying patients through this stage of their lives. Caregivers should encourage them to express their feelings freely, and reassure them that they can continue to lead as normal a life as possible despite the presence of the catheter. It may be useful to put them in touch with associations or support groups for patients with catheters or PEGs, so that they can exchange ideas with people going through the same experience.

• Care of patients with diarrhea, vomiting or incontinence
The care of patients suffering from diarrhoea, vomiting or incontinence requires special attention because of the significant impact these symptoms can have on their quality of life and general condition. These disorders, common in gastroenterology, can be the sign of a variety of pathologies, from gastrointestinal infections to chronic inflammatory bowel disease or the side effects of certain treatments. These symptoms, often a source of embarrassment, discomfort and exhaustion, require care that combines technical rigor, empathy and psychological support.

Managing diarrhea: rehydrating and preventing complications

Diarrhea, whether acute or chronic, results in a significant loss of fluids and electrolytes, which can rapidly lead to dehydration, particularly in fragile patients such as children, the elderly or those suffering from chronic illnesses. The first objective of care is therefore to compensate for these losses by ensuring that the patient is adequately hydrated.

The caregiver plays a crucial role in the assessment and management of diarrhea. They must monitor the frequency, volume and consistency of stools to enable the doctor to adapt treatment to the severity of symptoms. These observations are important in assessing the effectiveness of treatment, or in warning of complications such as severe dehydration, manifested by dry mucous membranes, hypotension, tachycardia or reduced diuresis.

Rehydration is essential, and can be administered orally or, in the most severe cases, intravenously. The caregiver ensures that the patient regularly takes small quantities of electrolyte-enriched fluids (oral rehydration solutions) to compensate for losses. If an infusion is required, he or she also monitors the correct administration of the solutions.

Diarrhea can also be associated with skin irritation, particularly in the perianal area, due to the acidic nature of stools and their frequent contact with the skin. The caregiver must be attentive to the patient's hygiene, carefully cleaning the area with mild products and applying protective creams to prevent rashes or ulcerations. If the patient is bedridden, it is also important to prevent bedsores, which can occur as a result of repeated care and the rubbing of sheets against weakened skin.

Finally, the caregiver must also take into account the patient's psychological comfort. Diarrhea, particularly when uncontrollable, can be a source of great discomfort, especially in a hospital setting. It's crucial to reassure the patient that these situations are handled with discretion and without judgment. Offering to help them wash or change their sheets quickly and sympathetically helps to reduce their anxiety and preserve their dignity.

Vomiting management: dehydration prevention and comfort

Vomiting, which is common in many digestive pathologies or as a reaction to certain treatments, such as chemotherapy, can be disabling and a source of great suffering for the patient. Like diarrhea, it can lead to rapid dehydration, but it can also cause considerable discomfort and lead to complications such as esophageal damage or electrolyte disorders.

Managing vomiting begins with careful observation of the symptoms. The caregiver must monitor the frequency of vomiting, its appearance (presence of blood or bile), and its onset (related to meals, treatments or spontaneous). This information is essential for adapting therapeutic management, including the administration of anti-emetic drugs prescribed to relieve the patient.

A key aspect of care is preventing dehydration. When vomiting persists, the caregiver must ensure that the patient receives regular hydration, often in small sips or intravenously if the condition so requires. Monitoring fluid intake and clinical signs of dehydration, such as a dry tongue or reduced urine output, is essential to avoid serious complications.

In terms of comfort, it's essential to help the patient maintain a position that facilitates the passage of vomit while reducing the risk of inhalation or suffocation. A semi-seated position is generally recommended, especially for bedridden or weak patients. The caregiver must ensure that the patient has an emesis basin or bag close at hand, and is quickly assisted if necessary. After each episode, it is important to clean the patient's mouth with water or a mild solution to avoid irritation of the oral mucosa and eliminate the unpleasant taste.

On a psychological level, repeated vomiting can exhaust and demoralize patients. Caregivers must be attentive to this suffering and show empathy. By explaining that solutions exist to relieve these symptoms, by ensuring a clean and soothing environment after each episode, and by encouraging the patient to express his or her fears, they help to alleviate anxiety.

Incontinence care: comfort, dignity and hygiene

Incontinence, whether urinary or fecal, is a major source of discomfort and loss of dignity for patients. This condition may arise as a result of general debilitation, neurological pathology or surgery. Managing incontinence requires a particularly delicate approach, where the aim is to preserve the patient's dignity while ensuring comfort and hygiene.

The first step is to ensure the patient's cleanliness, by regularly monitoring for signs of incontinence and promptly changing absorbent pads or soiled underwear. It is important that these gestures are carried out with respect and discretion, avoiding any comments that might reinforce the patient's feeling of discomfort. Hygiene care should be carried out using gentle products, especially for the fragile skin of bedridden patients or those suffering from skin disorders. Particular attention must be paid to preventing pressure sores in areas of prolonged contact with protective covers, especially the pelvis and buttocks.

The use of appropriate protection for the patient's condition is essential to guarantee both comfort and autonomy, wherever possible. For mobile patients, the caregiver can suggest discreet, easy-to-change pads, to enable the patient to retain a degree of independence. For bedridden patients, more regular care and monitoring of areas at risk of irritation are necessary.

Incontinence care also includes psychological support. This condition can be experienced as a real affront to dignity, particularly in adults who are losing control of their bodily functions. It is essential that caregivers adopt an empathetic and reassuring attitude, explaining that incontinence is a common medical condition and normalizing the situation. Offering discreet, proactive help, without waiting for the patient to request an intervention, helps to reduce anxiety and prevent embarrassment and devaluation.

3 Clinical monitoring and symptom management

- Observation of signs of deterioration (digestive haemorrhage, acute abdominal pain)

Observing signs of deterioration in gastroenterology patients, such as digestive hemorrhage and acute abdominal pain, is a crucial task that demands vigilance and responsiveness. These symptoms may indicate a serious complication, and require rapid management to avoid potentially fatal consequences. The nursing auxiliary, through its daily contact with the patient, plays a central role in this monitoring. They are often the first to detect the warning signs of deterioration, and their ability to quickly identify alarming symptoms is essential in preventing emergency situations.

Digestive hemorrhage: a sign to watch out for

Digestive haemorrhage is a frequent complication in gastroenterology, and can occur in a variety of contexts, such as gastric ulcers, esophageal varices, digestive cancers or chronic inflammatory bowel disease. It is manifested by the presence of blood in vomit (hematemesis) or stool (melena or rectorrhagia), or by discreet bleeding that may go unnoticed. The speed with which a digestive hemorrhage is detected directly influences the patient's prognosis, hence the importance of careful, ongoing monitoring.

One of the first signs of upper GI bleeding is hematemesis, i.e. vomiting blood. The blood may be bright red, indicating active bleeding in the esophagus or stomach, or darker, resembling "coffee grounds", a sign that the blood has been partially digested. The caregiver must be alert to any change in the patient's vomiting, and immediately report the presence of blood, even if it is in small quantities.

Melena, or black, tarry stools, is another indicator of digestive hemorrhage, generally linked to bleeding in the upper digestive tract (esophagus, stomach or duodenum). This symptom can go unnoticed if stool monitoring is not rigorous. The caregiver must be alert to any change in stool appearance, especially in high-risk patients such as those suffering from gastric ulcers, esophageal varices or taking anticoagulants. In case of doubt, it is essential to promptly notify the medical team to carry out further tests and confirm the presence of bleeding.

In some cases, digestive bleeding may be more discreet, but lead to a progressive deterioration in general condition. The patient may show signs of anemia, such as unusual pallor, severe fatigue, dizziness or tachycardia (increased heart rate), reflecting the body's compensation for blood loss. The caregiver, who is in regular contact with the patient, is often in the best position to notice these subtle signs and report them promptly.

Acute abdominal pain: a warning signal

Acute abdominal pain is another major symptom in gastroenterology, often associated with serious pathologies requiring urgent intervention. Whether related to intestinal perforation, pancreatitis, intestinal obstruction or mesenteric ischemia, this pain is often severe and sudden, and an important warning signal.

The first step in managing acute abdominal pain is to quickly assess its intensity, location and characteristics. The caregiver can ask the patient questions to better understand the nature of the pain: "Is the pain continuous, or does it come in waves?", "Is it localized to a specific area, or is it diffuse?", "Are there any factors that aggravate or relieve this pain?". This information is essential to help the medical team make a rapid diagnosis and guide further tests.

Severe abdominal pain, especially if associated with signs of peritonitis (rigid abdomen, nausea, fever), may indicate perforation of a digestive organ, such as the stomach or intestine, or severe inflammation, such as acute pancreatitis. In this case, the patient must be treated urgently. Caregivers must be alert to the rapid onset of symptoms and to changes in the patient's general condition, particularly if he or she becomes agitated, sweats profusely or has difficulty breathing.

In cases of intestinal obstruction, pain is often accompanied by vomiting and an absence of stools or gas. This type of pain, generally paroxysmal, may worsen over time, leading to visible abdominal distension. The caregiver should be alert to patient complaints of abdominal cramping or increasing discomfort, especially in patients with a history of abdominal surgery or inflammatory bowel disease, as they are at greater risk of obstruction.

In the case of mesenteric ischemia, due to reduced blood flow in the intestinal arteries, the pain is often described as very intense and out of proportion to the visible clinical signs. The caregiver may note that, despite the intensity of the pain, the abdomen appears relatively normal on palpation. This condition is an absolute emergency, as it can rapidly lead to intestinal necrosis.

The importance of communication and responsiveness

Faced with these signs of deterioration, responsiveness is crucial. Although not in charge of medical diagnosis, the nursing auxiliary plays an essential role in alerting the medical team quickly and accurately. As soon as an alarming sign is detected - be it digestive bleeding or acute abdominal pain - it is imperative to convey this information clearly and immediately. Observations must be factual and precise, describing the symptoms observed (type of bleeding, location and intensity of pain, changes in general condition), so that the doctor can quickly take the necessary decisions.

In addition to communicating with the medical team, the caregiver must also be a reassuring presence for the patient. These symptoms can be extremely distressing, and the caregiver's role is to remain calm, reassure the patient that measures are being taken, and provide comfort care while awaiting medical attention.

Preventing and anticipating complications

Careful observation of signs of deterioration should not be limited to managing emergency situations. As front-line professionals, orderlies also play a part in preventing complications by keeping a close eye on patients at risk. For example, in the case of a patient taking anticoagulants, monitoring for signs of bleeding must be stepped up, by observing the color of stools, vomit or urine, and remaining vigilant for signs of anemia.

For patients suffering from chronic diseases such as Crohn's disease or ulcerative colitis, monitoring abdominal pain and transit disorders (diarrhea, constipation) is essential to prevent a severe inflammatory flare-up or complications such as intestinal obstruction. By remaining attentive to the evolution of symptoms, the caregiver enables early management, thus limiting the risk of sudden deterioration.

- Stool, vomit and hydration monitoring

Monitoring bowel movements, vomiting and hydration is an essential task in gastroenterology, where these parameters often reflect changes in a patient's state of health. They are invaluable indicators for assessing the severity of a pathology, preventing complications or measuring the effectiveness of ongoing treatments. Caregivers play a fundamental role in this day-to-day monitoring, as they are often on the front line when it comes to observing and reporting any changes that may occur. Rigorous observation, combined with accurate transmission of information to the medical team, is crucial to ensuring optimal patient care.

Stool monitoring: a key indicator of digestive health

Stool characteristics (frequency, consistency, color) are crucial elements in the follow-up of gastroenterology patients. They provide valuable information on digestive function, the inflammatory state of the intestine, and may even indicate the presence of bleeding or infection. A change in stool frequency or consistency can signal a deterioration in the patient's condition, the onset of a complication, or the efficacy of a treatment.

The caregiver must be attentive to these changes, and gather precise information about the patient's bowel movements. For example, in a patient suffering from chronic diarrhea, the frequency of bowel movements may increase in the event of an inflammatory flare-up, as in Crohn's disease or ulcerative colitis. Caregivers should note the number of stools per day, their consistency (liquid, pasty, formed) and, if possible, their volume. These data can be used to assess whether the diarrhea is worsening, requiring a reassessment of treatment, or whether it is stabilizing.

The appearance of the stool is also very important. Black, tarry stools)melena) may indicate the presence of digested blood, a sign of upper digestive haemorrhage. Similarly, stools containing bright red blood (rectorrhagia) may indicate bleeding in the lower digestive tract, such as the rectum or colon. The presence of mucus in the stools, or very fatty, shiny stools (steatorrhea), may indicate a malabsorption disorder, requiring specific treatment.

In patients hospitalized for constipation or intestinal obstruction, the absence of stools must be rigorously monitored. In the event of prolonged constipation or obstruction, the caregiver should be alert to the appearance of abdominal pain, bloating or nausea, which may signal a worsening of the condition.

Monitoring vomiting: identifying complications and preventing dehydration

Vomiting is a frequent occurrence in gastroenterology patients, and can be a symptom of many pathologies, such as intestinal obstruction, gastritis, pancreatitis, or a complication of treatment (chemotherapy, antibiotics). They are also a source of rapid dehydration, especially if they are abundant and repeated. Monitoring vomiting is therefore a key parameter in preventing a deterioration in the patient's general condition.

The caregiver must observe and report on several aspects of the vomiting. Frequency is of course important: repeated or persistent vomiting over several hours requires special attention. The nature and appearance of the vomiting must also be noted. Vomiting containing bright red blood (hematemesis) is often a sign of upper digestive bleeding, while vomiting resembling "coffee grounds" suggests that the blood has been partially digested, revealing earlier bleeding in the stomach.

Bilious vomiting (green-colored, containing bile) may indicate a blockage in the intestine or a digestive obstruction, requiring urgent medical intervention. In addition, yellow or brown vomit may indicate regurgitation of intestinal contents, particularly in cases of intestinal obstruction.

It is also essential to monitor the patient's reaction to vomiting, especially if accompanied by acute abdominal pain, signs of dehydration (dry mouth, fatigue, confusion), or respiratory distress. Caregivers must be particularly vigilant with at-risk patients, such as the elderly or debilitated, in whom vomiting can rapidly lead to serious complications.

Monitoring hydration: a vital balance

Hydration is a vital parameter, especially in patients suffering from diarrhea, vomiting or fever, who may lose large quantities of fluids and electrolytes. Dehydration, if not detected and corrected promptly, can lead to serious complications, such as acute renal failure, confusion or hypovolemic shock.

Caregivers must therefore be alert to the clinical signs of dehydration, particularly in patients with significant fluid losses. These signs include dry mouth and skin, intense thirst, decreased urine output, excessive fatigue, dizziness or orthostatic hypotension (drop in blood pressure when standing). In elderly patients, dehydration may also manifest itself as disturbed consciousness or agitation.

Monitoring hydration also involves monitoring fluid intake, especially in hospitalized patients. The caregiver must ensure that the patient receives sufficient fluids, either orally or by intravenous infusion, depending on his or her ability to eat and drink. In cases of profuse vomiting or diarrhea, oral rehydration may be difficult, and rehydration fluids may need to be administered by infusion to correct electrolyte losses.

Urine monitoring is also a key indicator of hydration status. A decrease in urine volume, or dark, concentrated urine, is often a sign of dehydration. The caregiver must then inform the medical team to adapt management and, if necessary, implement more aggressive rehydration. In catheterized patients, diuresis monitoring (quantity of urine collected per hour) enables precise monitoring of hydration status and renal function.

Transmission of observations to the medical team

Monitoring bowel movements, vomiting and hydration is not limited to daily observation. It is essential that the caregiver transmits this information accurately and completely to the medical team, to enable appropriate care to be taken. The information gathered must be recorded in the care record and presented during inter-team communications, with details of the frequency, appearance and quantity of stools and vomits, as well as clinical signs of dehydration or hydration tolerance.

Clear, rigorous is reporting essential for adjusting treatments, such as the administration of antidiarrheals or antiemetics, or re-evaluating water intake according to changes in the patient's condition. It also helps anticipate serious complications, such as severe dehydration, renal failure or hypovolemic shock.

Psychological support for patients

Symptoms such as diarrhea, vomiting or dehydration are often a source of anxiety and discomfort for the patient. In addition to clinical vigilance, the caregiver must also provide the patient with psychological support. The repetition of these symptoms, particularly in a hospital setting, can affect the patient's dignity and quality of life, making them feel powerless or embarrassed.

It's important to reassure the patient that these symptoms are being closely monitored, and that solutions are being put in place to alleviate them. A benevolent, discreet and respectful attitude can relieve some of the anxiety these symptoms can engender. This also means swiftly dealing with uncomfortable situations, such as quickly changing bed linen in the event of incontinence, or offering to clean the mouth after an episode of vomiting.

- Pain and fatigue management

The management of pain and fatigue in hospitalized patients, particularly in gastroenterology, is a fundamental aspect of care, as both symptoms strongly influence their quality of life and recovery. Pain, whether acute or chronic, can be a direct sign of the underlying digestive pathology or the result of medical interventions, while fatigue is often related to the disease itself, to treatments, or to the side effects arising from them. The effective management of pain and fatigue relies not only on the administration of appropriate treatments, but also on a holistic approach that integrates psychological support, active listening and day-to-day accompaniment.

Understanding and assessing pain: an essential step

Pain is a frequent symptom in gastroenterology patients, whether related to inflammatory bowel diseases (such as Crohn's disease or ulcerative colitis), gastric ulcers, or post-operative complications. It is essential to understand the nature and intensity of the pain in order to adapt management effectively.

Pain assessment must be carried out systematically, taking into account the following characteristics:

- Pain **intensity**, often measured on a numerical scale from 0 to 10 (where 0 corresponds to no pain and 10 to unbearable pain), allows us to objectify its intensity.
- **The location of** the pain, which provides information on the organ affected and helps identify the underlying cause.
- **The type of pain** (burning, stabbing, pressure, etc.), which helps guide treatment.
- **The duration** and **frequency** of painful episodes, to monitor the evolution of pain.

The caregiver plays a key role in this assessment, asking the patient regular questions and observing his or her behavior. Some patients, particularly the elderly or children, may find it difficult to verbalize their pain. In such cases, indirect signs such as agitation, grimacing, muscle tension or crying may indicate physical suffering.

Medication-based pain management

Once the pain has been assessed, an appropriate management strategy is put in place by the medical team. This may include drug treatments, ranging from Tier 1 analgesics (such as paracetamol) to opioids for more severe pain, as well as non-steroidal anti-inflammatory drugs (NSAIDs) or antispasmodics, depending on the cause of the pain.

Although not in charge of prescribing medication, caregivers play an important role in administering and monitoring treatment. They must ensure that the patient receives the medication at regular intervals, as prescribed by the doctor, and that the treatment is well tolerated. If pain persists, or if side effects appear (such as nausea, excessive drowsiness or respiratory problems with opioids), it is imperative to pass on this information to the medical team, so that management can be adjusted.

At the same time, the caregiver should encourage the patient to freely express his or her feelings and comfort after the treatment has been administered. It's important to remind patients not to hesitate to ask for help if they feel even slight pain, as pain that is not properly managed can rapidly intensify.

Non-drug strategies for pain relief

In addition to drugs, non-pharmacological methods can be used to relieve pain. These techniques are particularly useful as a complement to drug treatments, or in cases where pain is moderate and manageable without systematic recourse to powerful analgesics.

Heat is often effective in relaxing muscles and relieving abdominal pain associated with spasms or cramps. The caregiver can offer the patient warm compresses to apply to the painful area, or help them take a warm bath if their condition allows.

Body **positioning** is also crucial in pain management. For example, a patient suffering from abdominal pain can be relieved by being placed in a fetal or semi-seated position, which reduces pressure on the abdomen and facilitates digestion. The caregiver can adjust the position of the bed, provide cushions or supports to help the patient feel more comfortable.

Relaxation techniques such as deep breathing, guided meditation or listening to soothing music can also have a beneficial effect on pain. They enable patients to turn their attention away from the pain, reduce associated anxiety and improve overall comfort.

Managing fatigue: a ubiquitous symptom

Fatigue is a common symptom in patients suffering from gastrointestinal diseases, particularly those with chronic conditions such as Crohn's disease, or those undergoing heavy treatments such as chemotherapy for digestive cancer. It can be due to a number of factors: the disease itself, malnutrition linked to poor nutrient absorption, chronic inflammation, or the side effects of medication.

Managing fatigue starts with recognizing its importance. Fatigue is not simply a normal consequence of illness, but a symptom that merits specific management. The caregiver must be attentive to the patient's state of fatigue, observing energy levels, ability to participate in daily activities (such as getting up, walking or eating), and mental state (mental fatigue, difficulty concentrating).

Rest is obviously central to fatigue management. The caregiver must ensure that the patient benefits from sufficient periods of rest throughout the day, without encouraging him or her to remain permanently bedridden. A balance between rest and light mobilization (according to the patient's abilities) is important to avoid complications associated with prolonged immobility, such as pressure sores or loss of muscle mass.

Adapting the environment to promote rest

To help patients better manage their fatigue, it's essential to create an environment conducive to rest. This can include adjusting the brightness in the room, reducing noise, and setting up a routine that includes moments of calm and relaxation. The caregiver may suggest limiting visits or scheduling care at times when the patient feels less tired, so as not to interrupt sleep unnecessarily.

Nutrition also plays a key role in managing fatigue. A diet adapted to the patient's needs, rich in nutrients and energy, is essential to compensate for losses due to malabsorption or frequent diarrhea. The caregiver can help to ensure that meals are taken in small, frequent portions, to avoid tiring the patient. They can also work with the dietician to ensure that the diet is adapted to the patient's general condition and specific needs.

Psychological support and active listening

Pain and fatigue are not only physical symptoms, they also have a significant psychological impact. Chronic pain can lead to anxiety, depression or feelings of helplessness, while prolonged fatigue can affect motivation and mood.

By being in regular contact with the patient, the caregiver plays an important role in providing psychological support. It is crucial to listen to the patient's complaints, to take into account their feelings, and to offer them a space where they can express their frustrations without feeling judged. Active listening, combined with reassuring words, helps patients to better accept their situation and understand that their condition is being taken into account.

Encouraging patients to take part in their own pain and fatigue management, by giving them tools for coping (such as relaxation or breathing techniques), also helps improve their sense of control and well-being.

4 Nutrition in gastroenterology: issues and particularities

- Dietary adaptations: fasting, specific diets (residue-free, high-fiber)

Dietary adaptations play a key role in the management of gastroenterology patients, as diet can have a direct impact on symptom management and the evolution of certain digestive pathologies. Specific diets, such as fasting, residue-free or high-fiber diets, are often prescribed to meet particular needs, whether to prepare the patient for an operation, promote healing, or reduce the symptoms of a chronic disease. Each dietary adaptation must be tailored to the patient's condition, while taking into account the nutritional requirements essential for maintaining overall health.

Therapeutic fasting: digestive rest and preparation for surgery

Fasting is a dietary adaptation frequently used in gastroenterology departments, particularly prior to certain surgical procedures or endoscopic examinations, such as colonoscopy. It consists in totally or partially restricting food intake for a given period, thus allowing the digestive tract to "rest", reducing the production of gastric juices, or facilitating observation of the internal walls of the intestine during examinations.

The aim of fasting is to limit gastric and intestinal contents to prevent the risk of complications during procedures, such as bronchial aspiration or contamination. For example, before a colonoscopy, the patient is asked to fast for several hours, or even an entire day, in addition to following a residue-free diet to cleanse the colon. This ensures a clear and precise view during the examination.

However, prolonged fasting can be difficult to bear for some patients, especially those already weakened by their illness. The caregiver plays an important role in ensuring that the patient is adequately hydrated, by offering water or oral rehydration solutions during the fasting period. They must also be alert to signs of weakness or hypoglycemia, such as dizziness, trembling or excessive fatigue, and alert the medical team if necessary.

The residue-free diet: relief for the intestine

The residue-free diet is prescribed in many situations, such as before a colonoscopy, or for patients suffering from acute inflammatory bowel disease (such as Crohn's disease or ulcerative colitis), or in cases of intestinal obstruction. The aim of this diet is to reduce the amount of fiber and food waste in the digestive tract as much as possible, in order to minimize irritation of the intestinal mucosa and facilitate transit.

Fiber-rich foods such as fruits, vegetables, whole grains, legumes and seeds are temporarily excluded from the diet, as they increase stool volume and stimulate intestinal transit. Conversely, low-fiber foods such as white rice, pasta, lean meats, eggs and low-lactose dairy products are preferred, as they are easier to digest and leave little residue in the intestine.

The no-residue diet is often perceived as restrictive by patients, due to the elimination of many fresh, nutrient-rich foods. The caregiver, in collaboration with the dietician, must ensure that the patient fully understands the objectives of this diet and the foods allowed, to avoid any confusion or frustration. It may be useful to offer appetizing alternatives, while respecting the restrictions, to maintain the patient's appetite and adherence to the diet. For example, clear soups, fiber-free vegetable purées or refined cereal products can be offered to vary the diet and avoid monotonous meals.

This type of diet must be followed for a limited period, as it can lead to nutritional deficiencies if prolonged, particularly in fiber, vitamins and minerals. It is therefore important to monitor the patient's nutritional status, especially if the residue-free diet is combined with longer restrictions in the case of a severe pathology.

The high-fiber diet: support for transit and intestinal health

In contrast to the residue-free diet, the high-fiber diet is often recommended for patients suffering from chronic constipation or functional bowel disorders such as irritable bowel syndrome. Fiber, found in fruits, vegetables, whole grains and legumes, plays a key role in regulating intestinal transit, by increasing stool volume and facilitating evacuation.

There are two types of fiber: soluble and insoluble. Soluble fiber, found in fruits such as apples, pears and citrus fruits, as well as in oats, has the ability to form a gel in the intestine, which slows transit and can be beneficial in cases of diarrhea. Insoluble fiber, found in wholegrain cereals, nuts and leafy vegetables, increases stool volume and speeds transit, helping to relieve constipation.

For patients suffering from chronic constipation, the gradual introduction of high-fiber foods can stimulate transit without causing excessive abdominal pain or bloating, which can occur if fiber intake is increased too quickly. The caregiver can play a key role in encouraging the patient to gradually incorporate these foods into his or her diet, and in helping him or her to follow the dietary advice given by the dietician. It is also important to remind the patient that hydration must be increased in parallel with fiber intake, as fiber absorbs water and a lack of fluids can aggravate constipation.

However, a high-fiber diet is not always appropriate, especially for patients with acute inflammatory bowel disease, where excess fiber can aggravate inflammation and pain. It is therefore essential to adapt the diet to the patient's pathology and progress.

Customization and adaptation of diets

Every patient reacts differently to dietary adaptations, depending on their pathology, general condition and food tolerance. This is why a personalized approach to diet is essential. For some patients, it may be necessary to combine several types of diet over the course of their treatment. For example, a patient suffering from Crohn's disease might benefit from a residue-free diet during an inflammatory flare-up, then a high-fiber diet during periods of remission to promote healthy intestinal transit.

The caregiver plays a central role in supporting these diets, ensuring that the patient understands the dietary instructions and monitoring his or her tolerance to these dietary adaptations. This includes observing the effects of the diet on digestive symptoms (such as diarrhea, constipation, abdominal pain or bloating) and passing on this information to the care team to reassess nutritional requirements as the pathology evolves.

The role of support and listening

Dietary changes can be difficult for patients to accept, especially when they are faced with restrictions that alter their lifestyle habits. Some patients may feel frustrated or limited by these adaptations, especially if they have to give up certain foods they enjoy, or if they have to follow a strict diet over a long period of time. Caregivers need to be attentive and supportive, to help them cope with these restrictions.

It's also important to involve the patient in the management of his or her diet, encouraging them to ask questions, express their food preferences wherever possible, and adapt their diet to make it more enjoyable, while respecting medical instructions. The caregiver's support helps to reinforce the patient's adherence to the prescribed diet, which is essential to guarantee the effectiveness of dietary adaptation and improve overall well-being.

- Enteral and parenteral nutrition: the caregiver's role in nutritional monitoring

Enteral and parenteral nutrition are often essential in the management of gastroenterology patients who are unable to eat normally by mouth due to their medical condition. These forms of nutrition help to meet essential nutritional needs and maintain optimal general condition despite the inability to eat. The caregiver plays a fundamental role in the nutritional care of these patients, ensuring not only the monitoring of medical devices, but also the patient's comfort and well-being throughout his or her treatment.

Enteral nutrition: feeding through a tube

Enteral nutrition involves administering nutrients directly into the digestive tract through a tube, when the patient is unable to eat normally, but the digestive system is still functional. This type of nutrition is indicated in a number of situations, such as after digestive surgery, in cases of swallowing disorders (e.g. after a stroke), or in patients suffering from chronic diseases such as Crohn's disease or ulcerative colitis.

Enteral nutrition can be delivered via different types of tube, such as the nasogastric tube (introduced through the nose into the stomach) or percutaneous endoscopic gastrostomy (PEG), where a tube is inserted directly into the stomach through the abdominal wall.

The caregiver's role in managing enteral nutrition is essential on several levels:

- **Monitoring probe function**: The caregiver should regularly check that the probe is correctly positioned and that the nutrition system is functioning without obstruction. It is important to monitor the patient's tolerance to nutrient administration, observing signs of comfort or discomfort (nausea, vomiting, abdominal pain) during and after administration. If discomfort is reported, or if complications such as tube displacement are suspected, the caregiver must alert the medical team immediately.

- **Maintaining hygiene**: Hygiene around the catheter is a critical aspect, particularly in the case of PEG, to avoid local infections. The caregiver must regularly clean the area around the catheter port with antiseptic solutions and ensure that the skin remains clean and dry. It's also important to watch for signs of infection, such as redness, swelling or the presence of pus around the insertion site.

- **Monitoring nutritional intake**: The caregiver must pay close attention to the quantity of nutrients administered and ensure that the patient receives the correct dose of nutritional solution according to the prescriptions. Monitoring the rate of administration is important, especially if nutrition is delivered over a long period of time, as an infusion that is too rapid can lead to nausea or abdominal pain, while one that is too slow may not cover the patient's nutritional requirements.

- **Psychological support**: enteral nutrition can be difficult to accept for some patients, who may feel a loss of autonomy or discomfort linked to the presence of a tube. The caregiver must offer psychological support, explaining to the patient the importance of this method of nutrition for his or her recovery, and accompanying the patient in his or her day-to-day life. Moments of dialogue and reassurance are essential to help the patient come to terms with this temporary or prolonged situation.

Parenteral nutrition: intravenous feeding

Parenteral nutrition is used when the patient's digestive tract is not functional or cannot be used, as in cases of intestinal obstruction, severe malabsorption, digestive fistulas, or after certain major surgeries. In this form of nutrition, nutrients are administered directly into the bloodstream intravenously, usually via a catheter placed in a large vein.

The caregiver's role in the management of parenteral nutrition is also central, although more focused on monitoring devices and observing the patient's general condition:

- **Catheter monitoring** : Parenteral nutrition requires the use of a central catheter (often a central venous catheter or an implantable chamber). The caregiver must ensure that the catheter insertion site is clean, dry and free from signs of infection. Particular attention must be paid to the hygiene of this area, as a catheter infection can have serious consequences, including sepsis. Daily monitoring helps prevent these complications and detect any warning signs (redness, pain, fever).

- **Infusion monitoring**: The caregiver must check that nutrients are being delivered correctly via the infusion pump. The flow rate should be checked regularly to ensure that the patient's nutritional requirements are being met. If the patient shows signs of discomfort, such as dizziness, accelerated heart rate or excessive fatigue, this may indicate an imbalance in intake (too fast or too slow) or metabolic complications associated with parenteral nutrition, requiring rapid intervention.

- **Monitoring metabolic complications**: Parenteral nutrition entails certain risks, including electrolyte imbalances and variations in blood sugar levels. The caregiver, in collaboration with the medical team, must monitor these parameters and be alert to the appearance of symptoms such as signs of hyperglycemia (excessive thirst, fatigue) or hypoglycemia (tremors, cold sweats). Early management of these imbalances is essential to avoid serious complications.

- **Hydration and patient comfort**: Although parenteral nutrition provides all essential nutrients, it can make some patients feel thirsty. The caregiver must ensure that the patient remains hydrated and, if permitted, offer small quantities of water or oral hydration solutions. In addition, because of the immobility imposed by the infusion, the caregiver must ensure the patient's comfort, by adjusting his or her position in bed, checking for pain or tension in the arm where the catheter is placed, and encouraging moments of gentle mobilization to avoid complications associated with prolonged bed rest.

Global nutritional monitoring: adaptation and personalization

Whether it's enteral or parenteral nutrition, nutritional monitoring must be rigorous and tailored to the patient's specific needs. Each patient reacts differently to these feeding methods, depending on his or her pathology, general condition and energy requirements. By being in constant contact with the patient, the caregiver is often the first to observe changes in his or her condition, whether in terms of tolerance to nutritional intake or signs of complications.

It is important for the caregiver to communicate regularly with the nursing team to adjust nutritional management according to the patient's progress. This includes monitoring weight, observing signs of malnutrition (such as fatigue, loss of muscle mass or the appearance of oedema), and keeping an eye on biological parameters that reflect nutritional status (albumin, electrolytes, etc.).

In addition, the caregiver must encourage the patient to express his or her feelings and needs. For example, some patients may experience hunger or discomfort despite artificial nutrition, while others may have difficulty accepting this form of nutrition. By actively listening to the patient and relaying this information to the nursing team, the caregiver contributes to personalized, patient-centered care.

Psychological support and assistance for patients

Enteral and parenteral nutrition can have a significant psychological impact on patients, particularly when prolonged. These forms of nutrition can be perceived as a loss of autonomy, or as a sign of the seriousness of their state of health. Caregivers play an essential role in supporting patients emotionally, by listening to their concerns and explaining that these methods are temporary or necessary for their recovery.

It's also important to reassure patients that they will receive all the nutrients they need to stay healthy, even if they can't eat conventionally. The caregiver must create a supportive and comfortable environment, ensuring that the patient feels cared for and respected in his or her needs, both physical and emotional.

Chapter 4

Participation in gastroenterology examinations and procedures

1 The caregiver and digestive endoscopy

• Preparing the patient for colonoscopy, upper endoscopy
Preparing the patient for a colonoscopy or upper endoscopy is a crucial step that determines not only the success of the examination, but also the patient's comfort and safety throughout the procedure. These endoscopic examinations, commonly performed in gastroenterology, enable us to visualize the inside of the digestive tract to diagnose pathologies such as polyps, ulcers, inflammation or cancer. However, for these explorations to be optimal and risk-free, it is essential to prepare the patient properly, both physically and psychologically. The nursing auxiliary plays a fundamental role in this preparation phase, providing instructions, supervision and support for the patient.

Physical preparation before a colonoscopy

Colonoscopy is an endoscopic examination of the colon, enabling direct visualization of the colonic mucosa using a colonoscope inserted through the anus. To ensure clear visualization and prevent food or fecal residues from obstructing the view, the colon must be completely empty. This is why physical preparation of the patient is essential.

The first step is to follow a **suitable diet** in the days leading up to the examination. In general, a residue-free diet is recommended 48 hours before the procedure, to minimize the presence of dietary fibers that could remain in the colon. The patient should avoid fruits, vegetables, whole grains and seeds, in favor of foods such as white rice, pasta, lean meats and dairy products. The caregiver plays a key role in ensuring that the patient understands these dietary instructions and follows them correctly to guarantee optimal preparation.

The day before the examination, it is common practice to ask the patient to **fast**, i.e. not to eat any solid food after a certain time, usually after dinner. He may, however, drink clear liquids such as water, broth, tea or filtered juices, in order to stay hydrated. The caregiver should check that the patient is following this advice and remind him/her of the importance of hydration, especially if laxatives are prescribed for bowel preparation.

Indeed, one of the most important steps is the administration of **laxatives** the day before or the morning of the colonoscopy. These laxatives, in the form of drinking solutions, are designed to induce complete evacuation of the colon. The patient must drink a large quantity of this solution in several doses. The caregiver is often present to supervise this phase, ensuring that the patient drinks the required amount and monitoring the effects of the laxative. It is important to reassure the patient, who may be bothered by the frequent and abundant diarrhoea caused by the treatment, and to remind him or her that these symptoms are normal and necessary for a successful examination.

It is also essential to watch for signs of **dehydration**, as laxative-induced diarrhea can lead to significant loss of fluids and electrolytes. The caregiver should encourage the patient to drink water regularly, while respecting dietary restrictions. If there are any signs of weakness, dizziness or fatigue, the medical team should be alerted.

Physical preparation for upper endoscopy

Upper endoscopy, also known as gastroscopy, is an exploration of the upper digestive tract, including the esophagus, stomach and duodenum. For this examination, physical preparation relies mainly on fasting to prevent food or liquids in the stomach from obstructing the view or causing aspiration risks during the procedure.

In general, patients are advised **not to eat or drink anything** for at least 6 to 8 hours before the examination. The caregiver must ensure that this instruction is followed and inform the patient of the reasons for this restriction, in particular to avoid any risk of inhalation of gastric contents into the lungs, a serious complication that can be avoided if precautions are followed.

If the patient is taking medication, the caregiver, in collaboration with the medical team, must check which can be taken before the examination and which must be temporarily suspended. Certain medications, such as anticoagulants or treatments for hypertension, may require specific adjustments to take account of bleeding or anesthetic risks.

Psychological support and patient information

Psychological support for patients prior to colonoscopy or upper endoscopy is just as important as physical preparation. These examinations can generate anxiety, especially if they are perceived as invasive or uncomfortable. Many patients fear physical discomfort, possible pain or loss of control due to sedation. It is therefore essential that the caregiver takes the time to inform the patient, answer questions and reassure him or her about the procedure.

A crucial aspect of support is to **demystify the examination** by explaining each step of the process. For example, the caregiver can describe the colonoscopy or gastroscopy procedure in a simple, reassuring way: "You will lie down comfortably, under light sedation. You won't feel anything during the examination, and you'll wake up quietly after the procedure". These explanations help the patient to prepare mentally and reduce anxiety.

It is also important to **create a climate of trust** by listening to the patient's fears. The caregiver should encourage the patient to express his or her concerns and ask any questions. If the patient is apprehensive about sedation or anesthesia, the caregiver can explain that the medical team is constantly monitoring vital parameters to ensure safety throughout the procedure.

In some cases, **anxiolytic pre-medication** may be proposed for particularly anxious patients. The caregiver, in liaison with the medical team, can administer these drugs and monitor their effect on the patient.

Material and organizational preparation

In addition to preparing the patient, the orderly is also responsible for **preparing** the **material** for the examination. He/she must ensure that the equipment required for the procedure is ready, that the examination room is well equipped, and that the patient is comfortably and safely seated.

The orderly must prepare the patient by asking him or her to wear **appropriate** clothing, usually a hospital gown, and to remove any objects that might interfere with the examination, such as dentures, jewelry or contact lenses. These simple gestures help to ensure that the examination runs smoothly and that the patient is kept safe.

* Assistance during the examination: patient set-up and anxiety management

Assistance during a gastroenterological examination, such as a colonoscopy or upper endoscopy, is a delicate moment in which the caregiver plays a key role. Their role is not limited to helping the patient settle in physically, but also includes managing the patient's anxiety, which can be significant both before and during the examination. Comprehensive, attentive care not only ensures that the procedure runs smoothly, but also reassures the patient and puts him or her in the best possible physical and psychological conditions.

Patient positioning: comfort and safety first and foremost

Positioning the patient prior to the examination is crucial to the patient's comfort and the success of the procedure. The caregiver must ensure that the patient is suitably positioned for the examination, while taking care to ensure the patient's safety and well-being. Every gesture must be performed with care and delicacy to reduce physical discomfort and minimize patient anxiety.

For a **colonoscopy**, the patient is generally positioned in the left lateral position, with knees slightly bent towards the chest. This position allows better insertion of the colonoscope and facilitates the device's progress through the colon. The caregiver ensures that the patient is correctly positioned and well supported by pillows or supports, to avoid any muscle tension or discomfort during the examination. It is also essential to maintain a certain degree of discretion to preserve the patient's privacy, especially when handling clothing and exposing intimate areas.

For an **upper endoscopy** (gastroscopy), the patient lies on his or her back or side, with the head turned to facilitate insertion of the endoscope into the mouth. The caregiver checks that the patient is correctly positioned on the examination table, with a pillow under the head for optimum comfort. He may also install a plastic mouthpiece (called a "mouth guard") to protect the teeth and prevent the patient from biting the endoscope during the examination.

Patient safety is paramount during these examinations. Before the examination begins, the caregiver must check that all monitoring devices are correctly installed, including vital signs monitoring (blood pressure, heart rate, oxygen saturation). This is particularly important when the patient is under **sedation** or light anesthesia, as he or she may not be able to communicate sensations effectively. The caregiver must also ensure that the patient has removed any potentially embarrassing objects, such as glasses, jewelry or dentures, to avoid any risk during the procedure.

Managing anxiety: essential psychological support

Anxiety is a frequent and natural feature before a gastroenterological examination, particularly for patients who have never undergone colonoscopy or upper endoscopy, or for those who fear unfavorable results. The caregiver plays a key role in managing this anxiety, providing personalized psychological support and ensuring that the patient feels safe and understood.

Creating a climate of trust from the moment the patient arrives in the examination room is essential. A smile, reassuring eye contact and a calm, soothing voice can help reduce the patient's stress level. The caregiver must adopt a caring and empathetic attitude, taking the time to answer any questions or concerns the patient may have before the examination. Good communication is essential: a simple, reassuring explanation of how the examination will be carried out, what sensations the patient may experience, and the approximate duration of the procedure, will help to remove some of the uncertainties that are often a source of anxiety.

Active listening is also essential in this phase. Some patients express fears about physical discomfort, pain or loss of control due to sedation. The caregiver should encourage the patient to verbalize these concerns, and remind them that the medical team is there to ensure their well-being throughout the examination. Explaining that measures are being taken to limit pain, such as the administration of analgesics or sedatives, can help alleviate anxiety. It is also important to remember that, even under sedation, the team constantly monitors the patient's condition to ensure that he or she is safe and comfortable.

In some cases, if the patient is **highly anxious, anxiolytic drugs** may be prescribed by the doctor prior to the examination to help the patient relax. The caregiver is responsible for administering these treatments and monitoring their effect on the patient. It is crucial to monitor the evolution of anxiety and to check whether the patient begins to relax before the examination.

Finally, **distraction** can be a useful tool for managing anxiety before an examination. Some departments allow the use of relaxation techniques, such as listening to soft music or guided breathing exercises, to help the patient calm down before the procedure begins. The caregiver can encourage the patient to practice deep breathing to reduce tension and nervousness, and thus promote a state of general relaxation.

Presence and support during the exam

During the examination, although the doctor is in charge of handling the endoscope, the caregiver remains close to the patient to ensure comfort and safety. He or she is often responsible for ensuring that the procedure runs smoothly, that the patient does not experience excessive discomfort, and that vital vitals remain stable.

If the patient is under sedation, the caregiver must monitor his or her state of consciousness and ensure that he or she responds correctly to stimulation. It is important to check that breathing is regular and that the patient is not showing signs of respiratory distress. If the patient is not fully sedated, the caregiver can speak softly to him/her throughout the examination, explaining the status of the procedure and reassuring him/her that it is running smoothly.

The caregiver must also be attentive to the patient's **tolerance** of the examination. For example, some patients may experience mild abdominal cramps or pressure sensations during a colonoscopy, while others may be bothered by the passage of the endoscope down the throat during a gastroscopy. In these situations, the caregiver should report any significant discomfort to the doctor, and ensure that the patient is as comfortable as possible.

- Post-examination monitoring and management of possible complications

Post-examination monitoring and management of possible complications following colonoscopy or upper endoscopy are crucial steps in ensuring patient safety and well-being. Once the examination has been completed, the caregiver's role is not limited to simple observation; it also includes proactive management of the immediate aftermath of the procedure, preventing complications and communicating with the medical team about any deterioration in the patient's condition. Particular attention must be paid to recovery from sedation, to clinical signs of possible complications, and to the patient's physical and psychological comfort.

Immediate monitoring after colonoscopy or upper endoscopy: recovery and safety

The first step after a colonoscopy or upper endoscopy is to monitor the patient closely in the immediate recovery phase, particularly if sedation or light anesthesia has been used. After these examinations, the patient is often drowsy or disoriented, due to the residual effects of anesthetic or anxiolytic drugs.

The caregiver must ensure that the patient gradually wakes up in a calm, secure environment. **Monitoring vital signs** is essential to detect any deviation from normal, notably by checking respiratory rate, heart rate, oxygen saturation and blood pressure. These parameters ensure that the patient is recovering from the effects of sedation, and that there are no signs of respiratory or cardiovascular distress.

It is also important to check that the patient quickly regains **clear consciousness** and is able to respond to simple stimuli. The caregiver should ask simple questions, such as "How do you feel?" or "Do you know where you are?", to check that the patient is gradually regaining contact with reality. If the patient shows prolonged confusion or excessive drowsiness, it is essential to prolong monitoring and report this delay in recovery to the medical team.

Postural monitoring is also necessary. The patient must be installed in a comfortable position, often in a semi-seated or supine position, to facilitate breathing and avoid falls or accidents linked to post-sedation disorientation. Particular attention must be paid to frail or elderly patients, who may recover more slowly.

Monitoring complications: signs not to be missed

Although colonoscopies and upper endoscopies are relatively safe procedures, some **complications can** occur, and early detection is essential to avoid serious consequences. The caregiver must remain vigilant throughout the post-examination monitoring phase, observing specific signs that may indicate a complication.

1. **Digestive bleeding**: After colonoscopy or upper endoscopy, there is a risk of bleeding, especially if biopsies have been taken or polyps removed. The caregiver should carefully monitor the color and frequency of the patient's bowel movements or vomiting. **Black, tarry stools** (melena) may indicate high digestive bleeding, while **bright red blood** in the stool or vomit may reveal active bleeding in the lower parts of the digestive tract. It is also essential to check for **signs of** acute **anemia**, such as marked pallor, dizziness, accelerated heart rate (tachycardia) or low blood pressure.

2. **Intestinal perforation**: Colon perforation is a rare but serious complication of colonoscopy. It often manifests itself as acute abdominal pain and a hard, tender abdomen, sometimes accompanied by fever or nausea. Caregivers should be alert to complaints of persistent or increasing abdominal pain after the examination, particularly if accompanied by signs of general deterioration, such as rapid breathing or general malaise. If perforation is suspected, the medical team must be alerted immediately, so that rapid intervention can be considered.

3. **Respiratory complications**: After upper endoscopy, patients may occasionally experience **respiratory distress** due to irritation of the upper airways or accidental aspiration of gastric fluid during the examination. It is crucial to watch for **signs of respiratory distress**, such as rapid breathing, difficulty in breathing or a drop in oxygen saturation. If such signs appear, the patient should be

146

immediately placed under reinforced surveillance, and medical intervention may be required.

4. **Urinary retention**: After sedation or anesthesia, some patients may experience difficulty in urinating. Urinary retention is more common in the elderly and in patients with prostate problems. The caregiver should check that the patient is able to urinate within a few hours of the examination. In the event of difficulty or discomfort, it is important to report the situation to the medical team to assess the need for treatment.

Patient comfort and reassurance

Once the acute monitoring phase is over, it is important to take into account the **patient's general comfort** and help him or her gradually regain well-being. The caregiver must ensure that the patient no longer experiences any adverse effects related to the examination, such as mild abdominal pain or bloating, which are common side effects after a colonoscopy. These symptoms can be alleviated by simple gestures, such as assisting with mobilization to evacuate residual gas from the intestine, or offering sips of water or lukewarm drinks once the patient is awake.

Psychologically, it is essential to **reassure the patient** that the examination will go smoothly and that there will be no major incidents. Many patients, still under the effect of sedation, may be disoriented or worried about the results of the examination. The caregiver can inform them that the results will be discussed with the doctor at a later stage, while explaining that the procedure went well. Gentle, soothing verbal support helps to reduce fears and promote a calm transition to the post-examination phase.

Outing supervision and post-examination instructions

Once monitoring is complete and the patient is stable, the next step is to prepare for discharge or reintegration into a care unit. If the patient is an outpatient, the caregiver must ensure that he or she is **accompanied** home **by a relative**, as sedation can impair the ability to drive or make clear decisions for several hours after the examination.

Caregivers also play a key role in **passing on post-examination instructions**. He/she should inform the patient (and accompanying person if necessary) of signs to watch out for after the examination, such as unusual abdominal pain, heavy bleeding or fever. The patient should be encouraged to contact the care team or seek emergency medical attention if any of these symptoms occur. In addition, the caregiver should remind the patient of post-examination feeding recommendations (gradual resumption of light foods and liquids) and activity restrictions (rest and no driving) for the hours that follow.

2 Participation in specific therapeutic procedures

- Assistance with nasogastric tube placement, biliary drainage

Assistance with nasogastric tube placement and biliary drainage is a crucial step in the management of gastroenterology patients. These procedures, though commonplace, require a rigorous approach to ensure patient safety and comfort, while minimizing complications. The caregiver plays a key role, not only in supporting the doctor or nurse performing the procedure, but also in ensuring the patient's well-being throughout. His or her assistance is not limited to the technical aspect, but also encompasses anxiety management and post-procedure monitoring.

Assistance with nasogastric tube placement: a methodical and humane approach

The nasogastric tube (NGT) is a device used to drain gastric contents, administer nutrients or medication, or decompress the stomach. It is inserted through the nose, then descends through the esophagus to reach the stomach. This procedure, although relatively simple, can be uncomfortable and anxiety-provoking for the patient, making careful support by the caregiver essential.

Preparing the patient: allaying fears and encouraging cooperation

Before inserting the catheter, the caregiver must ensure that the patient is fully informed about the procedure. The discomfort associated with insertion of an SNG can generate anxiety, especially in patients who have never had this type of device before. It is therefore crucial to take the time to explain to the patient the purpose of the probe, the duration of the procedure, and the sensations he or she may experience. For example, patients may experience temporary discomfort in the nose and throat, but it's important to reassure them that this discomfort is short-lived.

The caregiver can suggest breathing techniques to help the patient relax and reduce discomfort during probe insertion. Deep, regular breathing calms nausea reflexes and makes the procedure more bearable. It is also essential to ensure that the patient is in a seated position, with the torso tilted slightly forward, to facilitate probe insertion.

Technical assistance during the procedure

During catheter insertion, the caregiver assists the doctor or nurse by providing the necessary equipment (lubricating gel, air syringe to check catheter position, gloves, sterile compresses) and monitoring the patient. It's crucial to ensure that the equipment is sterile and ready to use, to avoid any interruptions during the procedure.

The caregiver can also help **stabilize the patient's head** to limit sudden movements that could interfere with probe insertion. While the probe is being inserted, the patient may experience a gag reflex, particularly when the probe passes through the back of the throat. It is therefore essential that the caregiver continues to encourage the patient to relax and breathe deeply to facilitate the passage of the probe into the esophagus.

Once the probe has been inserted into the stomach, it is necessary to check that it is correctly positioned. The caregiver can help at this stage by preparing an air syringe and a stethoscope to check that the probe is correctly positioned in the stomach (usually by injecting a little air into the probe and listening to the stomach sounds). Sometimes, an X-ray can be taken to confirm the position of the probe.

Positioning and securing the probe

Once the probe has been positioned correctly, **it** is important to secure **the probe** to prevent it from moving or coming loose. The caregiver ensures that the adhesive attachment is carefully applied to the patient's nose, without interfering with breathing or causing irritation. The caregiver should also check that the probe does not cause excessive friction or discomfort in the nostrils.

Assistance with biliary drainage: a more invasive and delicate procedure

Biliary drainage, whether internal (endoscopic drainage) or external (Kehr drain, T-tube drain), is a procedure designed to drain bile when the bile flow is obstructed. It is frequently used in patients with cholecystitis, gallstones or obstructive tumors. The procedure is more invasive than NGLS, and may require local or general anesthesia. The caregiver's role is to accompany the patient during preparation and ensure rigorous post-procedure monitoring.

Preparing the patient for biliary drainage

Prior to the procedure, it is essential to **prepare the patient psychologically**. Biliary drainage can be a source of anxiety, as it is often perceived as an invasive procedure. The caregiver must explain the procedure in simple, appropriate terms, and reassure the patient that he or she will feel no pain, especially if anesthesia is administered. It's important to answer any questions the patient may have, and to offer empathetic support to reduce stress.

The patient should be placed in a supine position, and the caregiver should check that the patient is comfortable before starting the procedure. As with the nasogastric tube, it is essential to ensure that all equipment is sterile and ready for use.

Assistance during the procedure

Although not directly involved in biliary drain insertion, the nursing auxiliary provides **technical support** to the physician by assisting with equipment preparation, ensuring hygiene and sterility of the environment, and monitoring the patient's vital parameters during the procedure.

In the case of **external biliary drainage**, the caregiver can help keep the surgical area clean, by disposing of the drained bile fluid into a sterile manifold, while ensuring that the drainage tube is properly secured to the skin. Monitoring the volume and color of drained bile is also an important task after drainage. This helps to ensure that the drainage is working properly, and to anticipate potential complications, such as drain obstruction or infection.

Post-procedure monitoring

After biliary drainage, monitoring is particularly important for **early detection of potential complications**, such as bleeding, infection or bile leakage. The caregiver must carefully monitor the amount of bile evacuated and the appearance of the drainage site. Excessive drainage, bile containing blood, or signs of infection (redness, swelling, pain) should be reported immediately to the medical team.

It is also necessary to monitor the patient's vital parameters after the procedure, especially if anesthesia has been used. The caregiver checks that the patient is recovering properly, that there are no signs of respiratory distress or severe pain, and that he or she can move without difficulty.

Patient comfort after the procedure is also a priority. The caregiver must ensure that the patient is comfortable, that the drain is secure, and that the patient's position does not interfere with the flow of bile.

Psychological support and follow-up

Whether it's the insertion of a nasogastric tube or biliary drainage, the psychological aspect must not be neglected. Caregivers must listen to patients, answer their questions and reassure them throughout the process. Some patients may be destabilized by the presence of these devices, feeling a loss of autonomy or discomfort. It is therefore important to encourage them to express their feelings, and to explain the next steps in their treatment.

- Care after digestive surgery (colostomy, intestinal resection)

Care after digestive surgery, whether colostomy or bowel resection, is crucial to ensure a good patient recovery and prevent post-operative complications. These procedures, often performed for conditions such as colorectal cancer, Crohn's disease or intestinal obstructions, have a major impact not only on the patient's digestive function, but also on his or her day-to-day life. The nursing auxiliary plays an essential role in this convalescence period, providing physical, psychological and educational care for the patient. Post-operative care must combine monitoring of clinical signs, management of devices such as stomas, and attentive support to help the patient adapt to his or her new condition.

Immediate post-operative monitoring: safety and pain management

The first few days following digestive surgery are crucial, as the patient is vulnerable to various complications such as infection, bleeding or digestive disorders. The caregiver, in collaboration with the medical team, must be particularly vigilant during this critical phase.

Monitoring vital parameters is a priority. Regular checks of blood pressure, heart rate, temperature and oxygen saturation are essential, to detect any abnormalities that might indicate a complication, such as post-operative infection (fever, tachycardia), or internal bleeding. The caregiver must also monitor the patient's general condition, ensuring that he or she is gradually recovering and showing no signs of deterioration.

Pain management is another central aspect of immediate care. After digestive surgery, pain can be intense, especially at the incision site. The caregiver must ensure that the prescribed analgesics are administered at regular intervals, while monitoring their efficacy and possible side effects, such as excessive drowsiness or nausea. Well-controlled pain promotes faster recovery, as it enables the patient to mobilize earlier and adopt postures conducive to healing.

At the same time, **monitoring the surgical incision** is crucial. The caregiver must check that the wound remains clean, without excessive redness or abnormal discharge, which could be signs of infection. Wound care, including regular dressing changes and maintaining hygiene around the operated area, is part of the daily routine.

Device management: ostomy care

After a colostomy, which involves creating an opening in the abdomen to allow stool to be evacuated through a collection bag, stoma care is a priority. An ostomy profoundly changes the patient's daily life, both physically and psychologically. The caregiver plays a central role in supporting the patient, ensuring proper management of the stoma and helping him or her to adapt to this new mode of functioning.

Ostomy care begins with rigorous monitoring of the appearance of the stoma itself. It should be pink to bright red in color, a sign of good blood circulation. Any change in color, such as blue, black or white areas, may indicate a blood perfusion problem, and should be reported immediately to the medical team. The caregiver should also watch for signs of infection or irritation around the stoma (the peristomal skin), such as redness, pain or abnormal discharge.

Changing the colostomy bag is a delicate but essential step. The caregiver must ensure that the pouch is watertight, to avoid leaks and maintain the patient's hygiene. He or she must gently clean the area around the stoma with suitable products, apply skin protection to prevent irritation, and change the collection pouch to ensure the patient's comfort and safety. The caregiver must also gradually teach the patient how to manage these changes himself, to enable him to regain a degree of autonomy.

Feeding and transit resumption

Managing feeding after digestive surgery is often a challenge, as the digestive system can be disrupted by the surgery. **Restoring bowel function** is a priority after bowel resection or colostomy, as it helps to assess whether digestive functions are returning to normal. The caregiver must carefully monitor bowel movements, the presence of gas, and the absence of severe abdominal pain, all of which are signs of a gradual return to normal bowel function.

In the first few days after surgery, the patient may be on **parenteral nutrition** (intravenous) or enteral **nutrition** (via a tube), while his or her digestive system readjusts. The caregiver must monitor nutritional intake and ensure that the patient is well hydrated, especially if transit is still irregular. Once oral feeding has been resumed, it is essential to start with a **light**, easily digestible **diet**, generally a residue-free diet, to avoid irritation of the digestive tract. The caregiver must ensure that the patient tolerates the reintroduced food well, without vomiting, diarrhea or pain.

Early mobilization and prevention of complications

Early mobilization is a key element of post-operative care, as it promotes blood circulation, prevents thromboembolic complications (such as phlebitis or pulmonary embolism), and helps the patient resume bowel movements. The nursing assistant, in collaboration with the nursing team, encourages the patient to get up and walk as soon as possible, depending on his or her abilities and general condition.

It is also important to **prevent pressure sores**, especially if the patient is bedridden for an extended period. The caregiver must ensure that the patient changes bed position regularly, and use anti-pressure sore mattresses or cushions if necessary. Careful monitoring of at-risk areas (heels, sacrum, elbows) helps prevent the development of pressure sores.

Monitoring for post-operative **complications** is also essential. In addition to wound infections or stoma-related problems, other complications may arise, such as internal bleeding, intestinal obstruction or digestive fistula. Caregivers must be alert to symptoms such as sudden and severe abdominal pain, vomiting, persistent bloating, or a prolonged absence of bowel movements, and immediately alert the medical team to any worrying signs.

Psychological support and therapeutic education

Digestive surgery, particularly colostomy or bowel resection, can have a profound psychological impact on the patient. The stoma, for example, can provoke feelings of loss of autonomy, embarrassment or shame, affecting body image and self-esteem. The caregiver, by listening to the patient, plays a crucial role in **psychological support**, offering empathic support and encouraging the patient to express his or her emotions.

It is also important to provide **therapeutic education** to help patients adapt to their new situation. The caregiver, in collaboration with the stoma therapist or nurse, can gradually teach the patient the daily gestures required to manage his or her stoma, or to resume a suitable diet after intestinal resection. The patient must be encouraged to regain self-confidence, to take ownership of his or her care, and to understand that, although his or her body has changed, he or she can return to a normal life.

The caregiver can also refer the patient to support groups or ostomy patient associations, which offer a valuable source of reassurance and information, especially for patients who find it difficult to come to terms with their new condition.

- Management of drains, complex dressings and wound healing

The management of drains, complex dressings and wound healing is a crucial stage in post-operative care, particularly after complex gastroenterology surgery. Whether placing drains to evacuate fluids, managing complex wounds, or monitoring the healing process, this care requires both technical rigor and attention to patient comfort and safety. The nursing auxiliary plays a key role in supporting this process, providing regular care, monitoring for signs of complications, and promoting optimal healing.

Drains management: prevention of complications and continuous monitoring

Drains are commonly used after surgery, particularly in digestive procedures, to evacuate fluids such as blood, bile or lymphatic fluid, and thus avoid accumulations that could lead to complications such as infections or haematomas. There are several types of drain, the most common of which are Redon drains, Kehr drains (used for biliary drainage), or Jackson-Pratt drains.

Monitoring the proper operation of drains

The nursing auxiliary plays a vital role in monitoring the proper functioning of the drains. The first task is to **regularly check the flow rate and appearance of the drained fluid**. Abnormally high volumes or unusual fluid colors, such as bright red blood or very dark bile, may indicate complications such as internal bleeding or biliary leakage. It is essential that the caregiver notes these observations in the medical record, and informs the nursing team in the event of any abnormality.

The drain's smooth operation also relies on **regular checks to ensure that the system is watertight**. If the drain is connected to a suction system (such as a Redon or Jackson-Pratt), the caregiver must ensure that the suction is active and that there are no leaks or obstructions. If the drain is blocked or not working properly, this can lead to a build-up of fluid in the surgical cavity, delaying healing and increasing the risk of infection.

Care around the drainage site

The site where the drain is inserted must be carefully monitored and cleaned. The caregiver must ensure that the skin around the drain remains clean and dry, and that there are no signs of infection, such as redness, swelling or purulent discharge. The dressing around the drain must be changed regularly, following strict hygiene protocols, to prevent local infections.

It is also important to **maintain the patient's comfort** by ensuring that the drain is properly secured and does not cause irritation or discomfort. The caregiver should help the patient adopt postures that minimize traction on the drain, which can relieve discomfort and prevent accidental dislodgement.

Managing complex dressings: rigor and meticulous monitoring

Complex dressings, often required after major surgery, are designed to protect wounds, promote healing and prevent infection. They may include absorbent dressings, vacuum dressings (negative pressure therapy), or antimicrobial dressings. Managing these dressings requires rigorous attention to wound evolution and patient comfort.

Changing complex dressings

Complex dressings must be changed under strict **aseptic** conditions to avoid contamination. The caregiver prepares the sterile material, ensures that everything is to hand, and reassures the patient before starting. The dressing is carefully removed to avoid damaging healing tissue.

Once the dressing has been removed, the caregiver **carefully examines the wound**. It is important to assess the color and appearance of the wound, and to watch for necrosis, signs of infection (redness, warmth, purulent discharge), or maceration. The wound should also be measured to ensure that it is gradually decreasing in size, a sign of good healing.

The new dressing is applied according to the specific needs of the wound. Hydrocolloid dressings, for example, are often used to promote moist wound healing, while vacuum dressings are used to stimulate the formation of granulation tissue in complex wounds. Caregivers must ensure that these dressings are applied correctly, without wrinkles or tension, to guarantee their effectiveness.

Monitoring wound complications

Complications of surgical wounds are common, especially in high-risk patients such as those suffering from diabetes, obesity or who have undergone major surgery. Caregivers must remain vigilant for complications such as infection, wound dehiscence (opening of the wound), or abscess formation.

If signs of infection appear, such as increased pain, fever or abnormal discharge, it's crucial to notify the medical team immediately so that care can be adapted, including antibiotic treatment or surgical debridement if necessary.

Cicatrisation: a process under surveillance

Wound healing is a natural process that takes place in several phases: inflammation, proliferation of reparative cells, and tissue maturation. This process can take varying lengths of time, depending on the patient's state of health, the extent of the operation and the care given to the wound. The caregiver makes a significant contribution to **optimal wound healing**.

Create an environment conducive to healing

A wound that is well cared for in a clean, protected environment heals more quickly and with fewer complications. The caregiver must ensure that the wound is always clean and remains free from further trauma. If the patient is mobile, **gentle** movements should be encouraged, and efforts that could compromise the integrity of the wound should be avoided.

The caregiver can also advise the patient on the importance of maintaining a **good nutritional status**, as wound healing is largely dependent on an adequate supply of nutrients, particularly proteins, vitamins and minerals such as zinc. For patients who find it difficult to eat properly, specific nutritional management can be put in place.

Healing monitoring

Monitoring wound healing involves **regular assessment of the wound's progress**. The caregiver should observe signs of effective healing, such as the formation of new tissue (granulation tissue), progressive wound closure, and the absence of pain or excessive inflammation. If the wound appears stagnant or signs of deterioration appear, it is important to alert the care team to consider adjustments in treatment, such as the use of specific dressings or more intensive medical support.

In some cases, complications such as **hypertrophic scars** or **keloids** may develop, particularly in patients with a genetic predisposition to these scarring anomalies. The caregiver, in collaboration with the medical team, can recommend specific treatments, such as massages or pressure dressings, to reduce the appearance of these scars.

Psychological support and patient education

The process of managing drains, complex dressings and wound healing can be both physically and psychologically demanding for patients. Caregivers play an essential role in providing **psychological support**, reassuring patients about the progress of their wounds and encouraging them to express their concerns.

It's also crucial to **educate the patient** about home care once he or she has left hospital, particularly with regard to the management of dressings or drains, if these are to be retained. Patients need to understand how to watch for signs of infection, change dressings if they are self-sufficient, and know when to seek advice if in doubt. Solid educational support helps to reduce patient anxiety and ensure uncomplicated healing.

Chapter 5

Communication and support for patients and families

1 Psychological support for patients

- Understanding the psychological impact of digestive diseases on patients

Digestive diseases, whether chronic or acute, have a major psychological impact on patients, often far more profound than visible physical symptoms. Beyond the pain, discomfort and functional disorders they cause, these pathologies affect the self-esteem, quality of life and social life of sufferers. Patients suffering from digestive diseases not only have to cope with frequent symptoms such as abdominal pain, transit disorders or fatigue, but also with emotional repercussions that can profoundly alter their mental well-being. Understanding this psychological impact is essential if we are to offer patients comprehensive support.

Chronic illness: an upheaval in daily life

Some digestive diseases, such as Crohn's disease, ulcerative colitis, irritable bowel syndrome or cirrhosis, are chronic and progressive. Living with a chronic disease means **constant adjustments** to daily life, both in terms of diet and lifestyle. These adjustments can create a sense of **loss of control**, as patients find themselves forced to modify their behaviors, often unpredictably as the disease flares up.

Chronic digestive symptoms, such as abdominal pain, frequent diarrhea, bloating or fatigue, are also often a source of **social embarrassment**. Patients may feel embarrassed at the thought of having to leave often to go to the bathroom, of not being able to eat what others eat, or of not being able to participate in certain social activities. This discomfort can lead to **reduced social interaction** and **gradual isolation**, as patients may prefer to avoid certain situations to avoid finding themselves in an uncomfortable position. This social withdrawal, often involuntary, can accentuate feelings of sadness and anxiety, and sometimes lead to depression.

Chronic fatigue, another frequent symptom of digestive disease, adds to this situation. Patients suffering from chronic inflammatory bowel disease, liver disorders or other digestive pathologies may feel constantly exhausted, even after long periods of rest. This fatigue makes it difficult to accomplish daily tasks, which can lead to feelings of **frustration** and **helplessness**, as the patient feels limited in his or her physical abilities. Fatigue can also impair concentration, affecting performance at work or school, contributing to a **sense of loss of** self-worth.

Body image and self-esteem: a deep-seated problem

Digestive diseases can also affect patients' **body image**, particularly in cases where surgery is required. Patients who have undergone procedures such as colostomy or bowel resection have to adapt to permanent physical changes, such as the presence of a stoma. These bodily transformations, although medically necessary, can be experienced as a loss of control over one's body and provoke a sense of **diminished dignity**.

The presence of an ostomy, for example, can be perceived as an invasion of privacy and social life. Many patients feel **ashamed** or embarrassed, fearing leakage or odour in public, which leads them to withdraw from social interactions or avoid certain physical activities. The impact on **sexuality** is also significant. Some patients may feel less attractive or fearful of others' gaze, which can lead to relationship difficulties or a loss of self-confidence in the intimate sphere.

For people suffering from diseases such as cirrhosis, digestive cancer or celiac disease, visible physical symptoms such as severe weight loss, abdominal bloating or jaundice can also affect their self-perception. The body becomes an object of constant surveillance, and every physical change can generate **anxiety** about the evolution of the disease, reinforcing a negative relationship with one's own body.

Anxiety about disease progression

Some digestive diseases are incurable and require lifelong care. **Fear of** disease **progression** is a major psychological burden. This anxiety can be particularly acute during periods of remission, when patients live in constant fear of a new attack or a worsening of their condition. This uncertainty about the future course of the disease can lead to a state of **chronic anxiety**.

What's more, the treatments themselves can have a negative emotional impact. Some treatments, such as immunosuppressants, steroids or chemotherapy, can cause unpleasant side-effects such as mood disorders, weight gain or sleep disturbances. Patients can feel **trapped between** the symptoms of the disease and the side effects of treatment, reinforcing their sense of powerlessness and inability to project themselves positively into the future.

Social isolation and fear of judgment

Social stigma is another important dimension of the psychological impact of digestive disease. Certain symptoms, such as flatulence, noisy bowels, frequent diarrhea or vomiting, are perceived as embarrassing or inappropriate in society. These manifestations, although involuntary and uncontrollable, can make patients feel **ashamed**. They dread the gaze of others and fear not being understood, or even being judged, for symptoms beyond their control.

This **fear of judgment** often leads patients to withdraw from certain social or professional activities, reinforcing isolation and misunderstanding. Even within family circles or friends, patients may find it difficult to explain their symptoms or to gain empathy, as these digestive disorders are sometimes trivialized or misunderstood. This **social isolation** can worsen the patient's psychological state, plunging them into a vicious circle where anxiety and depression feed on physical and social difficulties.

Coping strategies and the role of caregivers

Faced with the psychological impact of digestive diseases, it is essential to put in place **coping strategies to** help patients live better with their illness. Caregivers, including nursing assistants, play a crucial role in this process. Their **active listening** and **emotional support** can do much to ease patients' anxiety.

Caregivers need to listen to patients' **concerns** and **frustrations**. Sometimes, simply offering them a space where they can talk freely about their symptoms, fears or difficulties, without being judged, helps to reduce their emotional burden. Information and **therapeutic education** also play a fundamental role. Explaining to patients how to manage their symptoms on a daily basis, teaching them how to adapt their diet, or how to better organize their activities, can reinforce their sense of control and thus improve their psychological well-being.

Support groups and **patient associations** also play an important role. These structures enable patients to share their experiences with others experiencing the same difficulties, to feel understood, and to exchange strategies for living better with their illness. Speaking out in these settings helps to break down isolation and put symptoms into perspective in a supportive environment.

- Support for anxious or terminally ill patients

Accompanying anxious or terminally ill patients is a highly sensitive part of care practice, where attention is focused not only on the physical aspects, but above all on the emotional and psychological dimensions. Whether it's a question of relieving anxiety in the face of illness, or providing comfort at the end of life, the role of the caregiver is essential. His or her approach must combine active listening, empathy and benevolence, while respecting the patient's dignity and humanity in his or her final moments or in the face of growing anxiety.

Supporting anxious patients: listening and reassurance

Patients suffering from serious illnesses, particularly digestive diseases, often experience great **anxiety**, which may be linked to uncertainty about their state of health, fear of treatment, or anxiety about the future. This anxiety can manifest itself in various ways: agitation, insomnia, panic attacks, or even pain amplified by stress. The first step in supporting these patients is to recognize their anxiety and offer them a place to talk.

Active listening: essential relief

The caregiver plays a central role in **active listening**, which is often the first source of comfort for anxious patients. This involves being available, listening to their fears, without judging or minimizing their feelings. Many patients need to express their fears about the disease, their worries about treatment or their uncertain future. At such times, the caregiver must show that he or she understands these concerns and is there to listen, even if he or she cannot always provide precise answers.

Reassuring patients about the care they are receiving is also a way of alleviating anxiety. Patients may be stressed by heavy treatments, invasive examinations, or simply by their stay in hospital. Explaining in simple terms what's going to happen, reminding them that the care team is attentive to their well-being, and showing that steps are being taken to ensure their comfort can help ease these anxieties. The caregiver's benevolent presence can transform these stressful moments into moments of support, when the patient feels surrounded and understood.

Relaxation techniques and stress management

In addition to listening, the caregiver can help the patient manage anxiety by suggesting **simple relaxation techniques**. Encouraging deep breathing exercises, moments of relaxation, or even distracting activities such as listening to soothing music, can help reduce emotional tension. These techniques, though simple, often have an immediate beneficial effect, especially when practiced in a calm, reassuring environment.

If the patient's anxiety becomes too overwhelming, it may be necessary to offer **anxiolytic medication**, prescribed by the doctor. The caregiver, in this case, ensures that the patient receives his or her treatment, while continuing to offer human and empathetic support, as medication alone is not always enough to relieve anxiety.

Accompanying terminally ill patients: preserving dignity and offering comfort

Accompanying terminally ill patients is a particularly delicate and profoundly human mission. At this stage of the disease, the main objective is no longer to cure, but to provide maximum comfort, relieve pain, and enable the patient to live his or her last days or weeks in dignity, surrounded by benevolent care. The caregiver plays a fundamental role in this process, providing both emotional support and ensuring the patient's physical comfort.

Palliative care: pain relief and physical comfort

Pain relief is an absolute priority when caring for patients at the end of life. **Pain management**, through the administration of analgesics, opioids or other specific treatments, is essential to ensure that the patient does not suffer unnecessarily. The nursing auxiliary, in collaboration with the medical team, ensures that medication is administered regularly and according to the patient's needs. They are also attentive to the evolution of symptoms, adjusting treatments according to the time of day or the intensity of pain.

Physical comfort is not limited to pain management. It also involves meeting the patient's basic needs in terms of hygiene, nutrition, repositioning to prevent bedsores, and mouth care. Caregivers must pay particular attention to the way in which they carry out these gestures, taking care to act with gentleness and respect, especially when the patient is weak and has limited reactions. Every gesture, even the simplest, such as passing a damp towel over the forehead or adjusting a pillow, must be performed with attention to the patient's **dignity**.

Emotional support and a caring presence

Beyond physical care, support at the end of life relies above all on **presence**. A presence which, even if silent, is of immense importance to the patient and sometimes to his or her family. Terminally ill patients are often filled with **existential questions**, thoughts about the end of their lives, impending death or their past. Some want to talk about it, while others prefer to remain silent. The caregiver must adapt to these individual needs, remaining open to discussion if the patient feels the need, but also knowing how to remain discreet and respectful of moments of solitude.

In these moments, the caregiver often becomes a **landmark** for the patient, someone they can rely on in these last moments, whether it's holding the patient's hand, sharing a reassuring glance, or simply being present to meet their immediate needs. This support is particularly important when the patient is alone, or when the family cannot be present all the time. The caregiver then becomes a fundamental human link, able to bring a little serenity in the face of the inevitable.

Family support

Supporting patients at the end of life also includes paying special attention to their **families**. The suffering of seeing a loved one at the end of life can be very difficult to cope with, and the family may be overwhelmed by emotions of sadness, anger or guilt. The caregiver must show great empathy towards the family, offering them information on the progress of their loved one's condition, answering their questions, and reassuring them that everything is being done to ensure the patient's comfort.

In some cases, the family may find it difficult to accept the situation, and the caregiver must play a **listening and mediating** role, while respecting the patient's wishes if he or she has expressed specific wishes regarding the end of life. It is important to remain neutral and benevolent, accompanying the family in their anticipated mourning while maintaining a respectful framework of care for the patient.

Respecting patients' wishes and dignity at the end of life

One of the fundamental principles of palliative care is **respect for the patient's wishes**. Some patients express precise wishes concerning the treatments they do or do not wish to receive, how they wish to spend their final days, or even choices concerning their funeral rites. The caregiver must ensure that these wishes are respected, by ensuring that the patient is fully informed of his or her condition and options, and by facilitating the implementation of these decisions wherever possible.

Dignity is another central aspect of end-of-life care. Respecting the patient's dignity means maintaining a respectful attitude, preserving privacy during care, and ensuring that the patient is always treated with consideration, even when unconscious or very weak. This is achieved through simple gestures, such as covering the patient during care or speaking softly to them, but also through a humane approach that emphasizes the fact that every person has the right to respectful accompaniment until the end of their life.

2 Supporting families: a comprehensive approach

- Explain care and treatment steps

Explaining care and treatment steps is an essential part of the relationship between caregiver and patient. Understanding a patient's course of treatment enables them to better apprehend their care, to have a clear vision of what lies ahead, and to feel more confident about medical decisions. Clear explanations, tailored to each patient's situation and knowledge, are essential to establish a climate of trust and reinforce patient acceptance of care. Caregivers play a key role in this process, by explaining medical terms in layman's terms, clarifying the various stages of treatment, and ensuring that the patient fully understands the objectives of each intervention.

Preparing the patient: understanding the importance of information

The first step in explaining care and treatment is to prepare the patient, showing them the importance of understanding their care pathway. Many patients are anxious about the unknown, especially when it comes to their own health. Caregivers need to take the time to talk to patients, understand their fears and answer their questions.

For some patients, it can be difficult to assimilate all the complex medical information they receive at once. The caregiver must therefore ensure that the language used is simple and appropriate. It is essential to check that the patient understands what is being said. This can be done by asking the patient to rephrase the explanations in his or her own words, to ensure that he or she has grasped the essentials. This process is essential for reducing anxiety and fostering greater cooperation during care.

Explain diagnostic tests and first steps

When a patient arrives at the hospital or clinic with a health problem, the first phase of treatment often consists of a series of **diagnostic tests** to understand the nature and origin of the symptoms. These may include blood tests, X-rays, ultrasounds or endoscopic examinations.

The caregiver must explain to the patient what these tests are and why they are necessary. For example, he or she may explain that blood tests are used to check the patient's general condition and look for signs of inflammation or infection. They may also explain that imaging tests (CT scans, MRIs) enable doctors to visualize internal organs and identify any abnormalities. Describing these steps helps to reassure the patient of the usefulness of these interventions, and to reduce fears linked to procedures that are unknown or perceived as invasive.

For more technical examinations, such as colonoscopies or endoscopies, it's important to detail every step of the process. For example, the caregiver may explain that the endoscope is a flexible tube fitted with a camera that allows the inside of the digestive tract to be viewed, and that light sedation is often used to ensure the patient's comfort during the examination. By reassuring the patient about how the examination will proceed, it helps him or her to prepare better mentally.

Explain immediate care and management

After diagnosis comes the treatment phase, which can vary according to the nature of the pathology. Some patients will require immediate medical care, such as infusions, injections or specific medications, while others will be referred for more complex interventions, such as surgery or long-term treatment.

In these situations, the caregiver must explain the **immediate care** the patient will receive. For example, he or she can explain why an infusion is necessary, pointing out that certain drugs need to be administered directly into the bloodstream to act more quickly. He or she can also reassure the patient about possible side effects and the course of the procedure, such as catheter placement or preparation before surgery. This anticipation enables the patient to better understand what's going to happen, and to feel safer.

For more prolonged care, such as hospitalization or chemotherapy treatment, the caregiver needs to explain the **structure of the treatment**: how long it will take, what the steps will be, and what side effects or sensations the patient might experience. For example, in the case of chemotherapy treatment, the caregiver can explain that each session lasts a certain amount of time, that the patient will be monitored during and after the infusion, and that side effects such as nausea may occur but will be managed by appropriate treatments.

Explain the steps involved in surgical procedures

Once the decision to undergo surgery has been made, patients often need to be reassured and informed about every step of the way. Surgery can be a source of considerable anxiety, and it's crucial to provide clear, soothing information. The caregiver must explain the different phases of pre-operative preparation, the surgery itself and post-operative recovery.

Before an operation, it's essential to prepare the patient well, especially with regard to the importance of **fasting** before the operation, the administration of pre-operative medication, and the monitoring that will take place during anesthesia. The orderly can describe the operating room environment, the team present, and the steps that will follow immediately after the operation, such as waking up in the post-interventional care room. By providing these details, he or she helps the patient feel more at ease in the face of the unknown.

In the post-operative phase, the caregiver must also explain the **recovery** process, the care required for healing, and pain

174

management. For example, he or she may specify that drains or catheters will be fitted to evacuate post-operative fluids, or that dressings will be changed regularly to monitor the surgical wound. By specifying the care to come, the caregiver helps the patient prepare mentally and physically for his or her convalescence.

Explain long-term care and therapeutic education

In some cases, treatment doesn't stop at the hospital. Patients suffering from chronic diseases, such as inflammatory bowel disease, will need to continue their treatment at home. Caregivers play a key role in **therapeutic education**, explaining to patients how to follow their treatment and monitor their symptoms at home.

The caregiver must ensure that the patient understands the importance of **taking medication regularly**, explaining schedules, doses and any side effects to watch out for. They can also explain the signs that require prompt medical attention, such as persistent fever, severe abdominal pain, or a change in the appearance of stools or urine.

In the case of more complex home care, such as managing a nasogastric **tube** or **stoma**, the caregiver needs to explain the precise steps involved. He or she can show the patient or family how to change a colostomy bag, clean the stoma, or check the correct positioning of a catheter. This learning process enables the patient to gradually regain self-confidence and acquire a degree of autonomy in managing his or her illness.

Checking comprehension and follow-up

Once the care has been explained, it's crucial to ensure that the patient has fully understood the information conveyed. This can be done by asking the patient to repeat steps, ask questions, or even perform certain actions under supervision, such as changing a dressing or administering a treatment.

Follow-up is also an important part of support. The caregiver must remain available to answer any questions that may arise as the patient progresses through treatment. Knowing that someone is there to help reinforces the patient's confidence and ability to follow the various stages of his or her treatment.

- • Support loved ones in difficult decisions (palliative care, poor prognosis)

Supporting loved ones through difficult decisions, particularly in palliative care situations or in the face of a grim prognosis, is a profoundly human and delicate mission. These moments often mark a decisive turning point in the trajectory of a patient's illness, and families find themselves faced with agonizing choices. The caregiver, in his or her role as support and mediator, can provide invaluable assistance to loved ones, offering them a listening ear, comfort and clarity at a time often marked by confusion, sadness and uncertainty. Accompanying loved ones in these decisions requires not only an empathetic approach, but also the ability to communicate sensitively and provide a reassuring framework.

A grim prognosis: a shock for families

The announcement of a grim prognosis, when a loved one's illness can no longer be cured or stabilized, is often a traumatic moment for families. The reality of this news can be difficult to accept, and loved ones are often overwhelmed by intense emotions, ranging from disbelief to anger to despair. It's at this point that the caregiver takes on the role of emotional support.

One of the first steps is to **create a listening space** where loved ones can freely express their emotions and questions. The caregiver must be available, attentive and ready to accept the sometimes strong reactions that follow the announcement of a grim prognosis. It's essential to let loved ones express their fears, frustrations and misunderstandings without judgment. Often, the simple fact of being able to talk about their pain to a sympathetic listener can relieve some of their emotional suffering.

At such times, it's also crucial to **reassure loved ones** about the patient's care, explaining that even if curative treatment is no longer possible, continuous and attentive care will be put in place to ensure the patient's comfort. Families need to understand that palliative care focuses on quality of life, pain relief and respect for the patient's dignity until the end. By explaining these aspects, the caregiver helps **demystify palliative care**, which is often misunderstood, and provides a more reassuring framework for loved ones.

Decision-making in palliative care: an agonizing choice for loved ones

The decision to engage palliative care is often a complex and emotionally charged process for families. It involves recognizing that a cure is no longer possible, and accepting that support towards the end of life becomes a priority. This acceptance is sometimes difficult for loved ones, who may feel they are giving up the fight, "letting down" their sick loved one. The caregiver must be there to **facilitate this transition**, providing clear explanations and supporting the family's reflection.

The role of the caregiver is to **clarify the meaning of palliative care**, explaining that it is designed to support the patient in a caring way, to relieve suffering and respect dignity. It's important to show loved ones that palliative care is not synonymous with abandonment, but rather a new form of care, focused on the patient's well-being and comfort. Sometimes, loved ones need to understand that choosing palliative care is a kind of act of love, as it allows the patient to avoid invasive and exhausting treatments that would no longer be of benefit.

Caregivers must also ensure that their loved ones have all the **information** they **need** to make informed decisions. This means answering their questions clearly and honestly, taking the time to

177

explain treatment options, palliative care modalities, and what this means in practical terms for the patient and themselves. The caregiver can also accompany families during discussions with the doctor, helping them to ask the right questions and better understand the answers provided.

Supporting loved ones in the gradual acceptance process

Faced with a grim prognosis or entry into palliative care, acceptance is a gradual process. Loved ones often go through different emotional phases, from **denial** to **acceptance**, anger and **bargaining**. The caregiver must be a **stable point of reference** to accompany them through this emotional journey.

In the early stages, some relatives may be tempted to seek other solutions, other medical advice, or to insist that aggressive treatments be continued, even when the benefits are limited. At such moments, the caregiver must show **patience** and **understanding**, supporting the loved ones while tactfully reminding them of the importance of comfort and quality of life for the patient. This dialogue must be conducted with empathy, respecting families' need to feel involved and listened to, while guiding them towards a gradual acceptance of the situation.

As families come to terms with the reality of the situation, the caregiver can help them focus on ways to make the patient's last days as peaceful as possible. This can include simple gestures such as being present, listening to their wishes, or participating in the patient's care in collaboration with the care team. Encouraging loved ones to maintain a caring and loving presence with the patient helps them to feel useful, and to find meaning in these difficult times.

The caregiver's role in managing the emotions of loved ones

Those close to terminally ill patients or those suffering from an incurable disease experience a multitude of emotions, some of them contradictory. They may feel profound sadness, anger, guilt or helplessness. Caregivers must be attentive to these reactions, helping families to **manage their emotions** without feeling judged.

Some families express **anger** at the disease, at the medical team, or even at the patient. It's important to understand that these reactions often reflect their pain and their inability to control the situation. The caregiver must therefore welcome this anger with kindness, helping relatives to verbalize and channel it constructively.

Guilt is also a common feeling among families who, faced with the decision to stop certain treatments or move to palliative care, may wonder whether they have made the right decision. The caregiver must reassure them by explaining that the palliative care decision is taken in the patient's best interest, based on his or her state of health and suffering. By emphasizing that every effort is made to respect the patient's dignity and comfort, the caregiver helps loved ones understand that they have made a decision based on love and respect, not abandonment.

Finally, the caregiver must offer a **supportive space** where loved ones can freely express their fears, anxieties and sadness. It's often helpful to remind them that these are emotions normal, and that there's no need to hide them. By creating an environment where families feel heard and supported, the caregiver helps to alleviate some of the emotional burden they carry.

The importance of communication and time

In these difficult times, **communication** is essential. Decisions relating to the end of life or entry into palliative care often require several discussions before they are fully accepted. The caregiver must encourage open and regular dialogue with loved ones, ensuring that they have all the time they need to ask questions and express doubts. Each family has a different rhythm for accepting the reality of the situation, and it is important to respect this rhythm, while continuing to offer clear information and explanations.

It is also essential to maintain transparent communication between the various care teams and families. The caregiver can play a **mediating** role, facilitating exchanges between relatives and doctors, explaining complex medical terms, or clarifying practical aspects of palliative care.

Support for loved ones during and after the terminal phase

Supporting families doesn't stop with making difficult decisions. Once palliative care is in place, loved ones may need ongoing support to cope with the progression of the disease. The caregiver must be there to help them understand the changes in the patient's condition, to participate in care if they wish, and to **live** the last moments with their loved one **to the full**.

After death, the role of the caregiver remains crucial. They can **listen attentively to** the bereaved, help them through the first stages of grief, and direct them to support resources if necessary, such as psychologists or discussion groups.

3 Handling difficult situations

- Anger attacks, refusal of care: how to react?

Angry outbursts and refusal of care are delicate situations with which caregivers, and in particular orderlies, may be confronted in their daily work. These reactions often reflect deep psychological distress, a sense of powerlessness or a need to regain some control over a medical situation perceived as oppressive. In the face of such behavior, it is essential to react with empathy, calm and professionalism, to relieve the tension and re-establish a climate of trust with the patient. The aim is not only to manage the crisis, but also to understand its origins, provide appropriate solutions, and enable the patient to regain a degree of serenity.

Understanding the origins of tantrums and refusal of care

Temper tantrums and refusal of care are often emotionally charged reactions. Behind these behaviors, there are usually deep-rooted causes which it is essential to understand in order to react appropriately.

In many cases, anger can be the result of a **feeling of powerlessness** in the face of illness or a medical situation. Patients, faced with serious diagnoses or heavy treatments, may feel a loss of control over their own bodies and the decisions being made on their behalf. This can lead to outbursts of anger directed at caregivers, who are seen as the "enforcers" of medical decisions.

Refusing care, on the other hand, can be a way for patients to **regain control** in a situation where they feel powerless. By refusing a treatment, examination or procedure, the patient reaffirms his or her ability to make decisions about his or her own body, even if these decisions run counter to what is recommended by caregivers.

It's also important to consider that these reactions may be linked to **deep-seated fear**. Anger may conceal anxiety about pain, fear of the unknown, or worry about the outcome of treatment. Refusal of treatment may also be motivated by fear of side-effects, additional suffering or deterioration in health.

Reacting with calm and empathy: the importance of de-escalation

The first rule when faced with a tantrum or refusal of care is to **remain calm**. It's vital not to react with irritation or impatience, even if the situation may be difficult to handle at the time. When faced with a patient's anger, the caregiver's reaction must be focused on appeasement.

Physical posture plays an important role. It's best to position yourself at the patient's level, avoiding abrupt gestures or attitudes perceived as dominant. A calm, composed voice, sympathetic eye contact and attentive listening are essential to resolving the situation. Showing the patient that he or she is being heard and taken seriously is the first step in reducing the intensity of his or her anger.

Active listening is one of the keys to defusing crises. Rather than immediately trying to convince the patient to accept care, it's important to give them the space to express their anger or concerns. Patients need to feel they can speak freely, without being interrupted or judged. This often helps to release some of the accumulated tension and to better understand the reasons for the patient's reaction.

It can be helpful to **rephrase** the patient's words to show that you've understood how he or she feels. For example, "I understand that you feel angry because you feel you're not being listened to enough" or "I can see that this situation is difficult for you, and it's normal to be worried". This reformulation allows the patient to feel validated in his or her emotions, which can help to calm the situation.

Seeking to understand the root cause of refusal of care

When a patient refuses care or treatment, it's essential to understand why. The caregiver, as the front line in the relationship with the patient, can play a key role in identifying the **sources of resistance**. These are often unexpressed fears, a lack of understanding of the treatment, or a desire to regain control.

One strategy is to **ask open-ended questions** to encourage the patient to explain their refusal: "Can you tell me what worries you about this care?", "Is it the procedure that scares you?" or "Is there anything you'd like to understand better about this treatment?". These questions explore the underlying reasons for refusing care, while showing that the caregiver is trying to understand the patient's point of view.

Once the reasons for refusal have been identified, it becomes easier to offer **reassuring explanations** or propose **alternatives** that respect the patient's concerns. For example, if a patient refuses a blood test for fear of pain, he or she may be reassured by the application of a local anaesthetic. If the fear stems from a lack of understanding of the side-effects of a treatment, clear, detailed explanations can help to overcome reluctance. The caregiver can then play the role of **educator**, explaining the benefits of treatment and answering the patient's questions.

Propose compromises while respecting patient autonomy

When faced with a refusal of care, it is essential to remember that the patient retains his or her **autonomy** and the right to make decisions concerning his or her health. However, it is possible to find **compromises** to avoid a total breakdown in the care relationship. The caregiver may, for example, suggest postponing the treatment, or carrying it out under conditions that better respect the patient's needs or concerns.

The idea is to involve the patient in decisions concerning his or her care, rather than imposing treatment. For example, if a patient refuses a nasogastric tube, it can be helpful to discuss alternative options, giving them time to think and ask questions. The caregiver can also ask the patient what they would like or what would make them more comfortable: "What can I do to make this care more bearable for you?".

Involving the patient in the decision-making process enables him or her to **regain a form of control**, which can sometimes be enough to ease resistance and re-establish a climate of trust. This constant dialogue between caregiver and patient is a powerful way of breaking down blockages.

Preventing temper tantrums: working in anticipation

While it's impossible to avoid all tantrums or refusals of care, they can often be **prevented by** anticipating the patient's needs and concerns. **Clear, ongoing communication** helps to reassure patients throughout their care.

Explaining medical procedures in advance, giving details of what the patient should expect, and answering questions even before they are raised, are all ways of avoiding misunderstandings and reducing anxiety. For example, before a potentially painful procedure, the caregiver can anticipate reactions by explaining precisely how it will be carried out, and suggesting ways of easing discomfort (such as local anaesthetic or distraction).

It's also essential to be **alert to the warning signs** of a temper tantrum. If a patient begins to show signs of impatience, agitation or frustration, the caregiver can intervene beforehand, taking a moment to talk with the patient, understand what's bothering him/her and adjust care accordingly.

Calling on the care team for collective support

In some situations, angry outbursts or refusal of care can be particularly complex and difficult to manage alone. It's important to recognize when it's necessary to **call on the care team** for collective support. Sometimes, additional medical advice or the intervention of a psychologist can help resolve a blocked situation.

The caregiver should not hesitate to share his or her observations with the team, to suggest adjustments in care, or to seek advice if the patient continues to refuse care despite several attempts at dialogue.

• Managing death in the gastroenterology department: a human and professional approach

Dealing with death in the gastroenterology department is an often difficult, but inescapable reality for care teams. The loss of a patient, whether expected or sudden, raises complex emotions for both family and nursing staff. It requires an approach that is both humane and professional, where compassion, respect and support are essential. As a caregiver, the role is not limited to the technical aspects of post-mortem care, but also includes accompanying families at a time of great vulnerability, while ensuring that a dignified and respectful environment is maintained for the deceased.

Accompaniment to the end: the patient's last moments

In gastroenterology departments, some patients are cared for in the terminal phase of their illness, as in the case of advanced digestive cancers, irreversible cirrhosis or other serious pathologies. When the end of life approaches, the caregiver has a crucial role to play in accompanying the patient in his or her final moments. The human and professional approach is to ensure that the patient is surrounded by compassionate care, focused on his or her comfort and dignity.

Palliative care, often implemented for patients at the end of life, is primarily aimed at relieving pain and troublesome symptoms, while respecting the patient's wishes. The caregiver plays a key role in providing comfort care, ensuring that the patient is comfortable, that pain is controlled and that hygiene is maintained. At this stage, simple gestures such as moistening the patient's lips, readjusting the pillow, or maintaining visual and verbal contact, even if the patient is unconscious, are essential to show the humanity and respect that the patient deserves until his or her last moments.

Accompanying the last moments also implies a **silent** but reassuring **presence**, even when the patient can no longer interact. The caregiver can ensure that loved ones have an intimate moment with the patient, uninterrupted, and be on hand to respond to any needs or concerns. Simply being there, available, can offer comfort to the family at this painful time.

Announcing a death: supporting loved ones with empathy

The announcement of a death is an extremely sensitive moment, often marked by shock and sadness for families. When a patient dies, the caregiver's priority is to ensure that **communication with next of kin** is clear and respectful. Although the official announcement of death is usually made by a doctor, the caregiver is often on hand to support families before, during and after the announcement.

The first step is to **create a suitable environment** for this announcement. It's important to offer loved ones a private, quiet space where they can receive the news without being exposed to outside scrutiny or the hustle and bustle of the hospital. The caregiver can prepare the family for this moment, by welcoming them with kindness and offering them moral support.

Once the death has been announced, the reactions of loved ones can vary greatly: some may remain silent, others may cry, or express their grief through gestures or angry words. The caregiver must remain **open to all these reactions**, giving them space to grieve, while offering a comforting presence. It is often helpful to offer loved ones the opportunity to stay with the deceased if they wish, while ensuring that the patient's privacy and dignity are respected.

The caregiver can also provide families with practical information on the next steps to be taken (administrative formalities, contacts with the funeral service), while taking care not to rush this moment of contemplation. It's important to give the family time to say goodbye to the deceased, without imposing any pace or constraints.

Post-mortem care: respect and dignity for the deceased

After death, one of the caregiver's main responsibilities is to care for the patient's body in a way that preserves its dignity. **Post-mortem care** is a highly symbolic act, which must be carried out with care and respect. It involves preparing the body for the visit of relatives, or for transfer to the mortuary, while taking care to respect the wishes of the patient and his or her family.

The first step is to **groom the deceased** gently, washing the body and dressing it appropriately. The caregiver must ensure that these gestures are carried out in a calm and dignified manner, bearing in mind that respect for the body is a form of homage to the patient. This includes closing the eyes, positioning the arms naturally, and covering the body with a clean sheet.

If relatives wish to see the deceased after post-mortem care, it is essential to ensure that the presentation is **soothing**. The caregiver can take care to explain to families what to expect, while offering private moments for contemplation. Loved ones can sometimes be upset by the physical change in the deceased, and it's important to stay close by to support them through this ordeal.

Supporting care teams in bereavement

The death of a patient can also affect the care team, especially if the patient has been cared for over a long period or if personal bonds have been formed. The caregiver, as a member of this team, may feel sadness or a sense of loss, particularly when the death is difficult or unexpected. It's important that caregivers can also **express their own grief** and find ways of coping with these trying times.

Within teams, it can be useful to set up a **time for talking** after a death, to enable everyone to express their feelings. This sharing can strengthen team cohesion and help overcome the emotional burden. The caregiver, although often perceived as the one who must reassure and support, may also need this mutual support. It is essential not to minimize the emotional impact of a patient's death on the nursing staff.

Management of administrative procedures and relations with the family

In addition to providing emotional support, the caregiver is also responsible for **coordinating the administrative procedures** required after a death. This includes liaising with funeral services, managing the deceased's personal effects, and transmitting the necessary documents to the family to organize the funeral.

Families, often in a state of shock, can be overwhelmed by the number of steps to take after the loss of a loved one. The caregiver can play a key role in **clarifying the steps** to be taken, providing simple, practical information, and directing the family to the right people or services. It's important to adopt a patient, caring attitude, respecting the family's time and avoiding imposing hasty decisions.

Taking care of yourself as a caregiver

Dealing with death repeatedly can be trying, and it's crucial that caregivers take care of their **mental and emotional health**. Caregivers are often on the front line of suffering and loss, and this can generate a build-up of stress or sadness. It's essential to recognize this emotional burden and find ways to manage it, whether through discussions with colleagues, debriefing sessions after a death, or relaxation techniques.

Healthcare institutions can also offer **psychological support** to care teams, particularly in departments where deaths are frequent. It's important that caregivers don't hesitate to use these resources to prevent burnout or feelings of overwhelm in the face of death.

Chapter 6

The specific challenges of being a gastroenterology orderly

1 Physical challenges: a demanding profession

- Management of heavy physical care)patient mobilization, complex hygiene care)

The management of heavy physical care, such as patient mobilization or complex hygiene care, is an essential task in the care of hospitalized patients, particularly in gastroenterology. This care is particularly important for patients who are bedridden, suffering from serious illnesses, or who have undergone major surgery. It requires not only technical skills, but also a human approach that places the patient's comfort, dignity and well-being at the heart of the care provided. The nursing auxiliary plays a fundamental role in this care, ensuring that the care provided is adapted to the patient's abilities and limitations.

Patient mobilization: preserving mobility and preventing complications

Mobilizing patients is a crucial aspect of heavy physical care, especially for those who are bedridden for long periods. Prolonged immobility can lead to complications such as pressure sores, respiratory disorders, urinary tract infections and thrombosis. Regular mobilization helps prevent these complications and maintain muscle tone.

Adapting mobilization to the patient's condition

Every patient has different physical capabilities, depending on his or her state of health, age, level of pain, and the procedures he or she has undergone. It is therefore essential to adapt mobilization techniques to each patient's specific needs. For example, a patient who has just undergone abdominal surgery will have difficulty getting up or moving around on his own, and it will be necessary to help him adopt postures that limit tension on the operated area.

Before any mobilization, it is essential to assess the patient's condition and **inform** him or her **of** what is to be done. This reduces anxiety and encourages cooperation. The caregiver must also ensure that **handling techniques** protect both patient and caregiver, using ergonomic postures and, where possible, technical aids (such as patient lifts or sliding sheets) to avoid any risk of injury.

Mobilization can be as simple as **changing position** in bed, turning the patient from side to side to avoid pressure points, or helping the patient to sit up on the edge of the bed to stimulate blood circulation. These gestures may seem minor, but they have a major impact on patient comfort and the prevention of complications associated with prolonged bed rest.

Encouraging independent mobility

Wherever possible, it's important to encourage patients to participate in their own mobilization. Even if the patient is weak, helping him or her to make small movements on their own, such as pushing with the feet or holding onto the bed frame, promotes rehabilitation and independence. The caregiver must remain close by to ensure the patient's safety and guide his or her movements, but it is essential to give the patient the space he or she needs to become actively involved in his or her own care.

For patients able to stand up with assistance, the caregiver can **accompany** them **to walk**, providing balance support, or using a walker or cane. These moments of active mobilization are essential for stimulating circulation, preventing the onset of venous thrombosis, and restoring patients' confidence in their physical abilities.

Complex hygiene care: maintaining patient dignity and comfort

Hygiene care is another important aspect of heavy physical care. Some patients, because of their state of health or immobility, can no longer take care of their hygiene independently. In such cases, the caregiver must intervene to provide this care, while preserving the patient's dignity.

Bedtime grooming: a delicate but necessary task

For patients who are bedridden and unable to get up, washing in bed is a crucial moment, not only for maintaining **good** personal **hygiene**, but also for preventing skin infections, bedsores and discomfort due to perspiration or the accumulation of body secretions. Washing in bed must be carried out delicately, ensuring that the patient does not feel vulnerable or exposed.

Before starting to wash, it is essential to **prepare the** necessary **equipment** (gloves, towels, basin of warm water, mild soap, bed protector) and to **inform the patient of** each step. Care should be performed progressively, covering unwashed parts of the body to maintain warmth and privacy.

Caregivers must ensure that **sensitive areas** such as skin folds, armpits, perineum and areas where medical devices are present (probes, drains, dressings) are thoroughly cleaned and dried. This care reduces the risk of infection and skin irritation. **Discretion** and communication throughout the care process ensure that patients feel comfortable and respected, despite their dependency.

Care of incontinent patients

The management of incontinence, whether urinary or fecal, is part of complex hygiene care, particularly in patients suffering from digestive diseases or in post-operative care. Incontinence can be experienced as a loss of autonomy and an affront to dignity, so it's crucial that this care is carried out with the utmost **delicacy** and **empathy**.

Regularly changing pads, ensuring that the patient's skin is thoroughly cleansed and moisturized after each change, and using appropriate care products to avoid irritation are all essential gestures. Caregivers must also be alert to **signs of irritation** or maceration, which can lead to skin infections or bedsores. This care must be carried out quickly and efficiently, while explaining each gesture to the patient so that he or she does not feel infantilized or devalued.

Perineum and ostomy care

Patients who have undergone digestive surgery, such as a colostomy, require special hygiene care, particularly at the stoma. Stoma management requires **technical precision** and special attention to avoid local complications (infection, skin irritation).

The caregiver must master the technical gestures required to **change ostomy pouches**, gently clean the skin around the stoma, and apply appropriate skin protection. This care also provides an opportunity to observe the peristomal skin for any abnormalities or irritation requiring medical intervention.

As with all hygiene care, it's essential to **respect** patients' **privacy** and reassure them about the progress of their care. The stoma can be a source of anxiety for patients, particularly when they have to adapt to it. The caregiver plays a key role in providing **psychological support**, explaining each stage of care and helping the patient to accept this new reality.

Mouth care, pressure sore prevention and skin monitoring

Long-term bedridden patients, especially those under sedation or suffering from serious illnesses, also require **specific mouth care**. Oral hygiene helps prevent infections (such as mycosis or gingivitis) and contributes to the patient's general comfort, notably by reducing dry mouth or unpleasant odours.

At the same time, pressure sore prevention is a priority for immobilized patients. This means **regularly changing the position of** bedridden patients, using anti-pressure sore mattresses or cushions, and checking the condition of the skin on a daily basis, particularly in high-risk areas (heels, sacrum, elbows).

The caregiver must be alert to **signs of redness** or skin lesions, which may indicate excessive pressure or poorly distributed pressure points. Preventing pressure sores is a care task in its own right, requiring constant monitoring, combined with good hygiene and skin moisturizing.

Respecting patient dignity throughout care

In all heavy physical care, from mobilization to complex hygiene care, the main objective is to **preserve the patient's dignity**. Every gesture must be carried out with respect, taking care to inform the patient and respect his or her privacy.

The role of the caregiver is to combine **technical skill** with **empathy**, so that even the most invasive or uncomfortable care is carried out in a climate of trust and serenity. Respecting the patient's rhythm, adapting procedures to his or her tolerance, and taking into account his or her physical and emotional needs are the cornerstones of successful care.

- Fatigue due to shift work and emotional strain

Fatigue linked to shifting working hours and emotional strain is an ever-present reality for caregivers, especially those working in demanding departments such as gastroenterology. Working shifts, nights or weekends, combined with the heavy emotional burden inherent in caring for often seriously ill patients, can lead to physical and mental exhaustion. This fatigue, if not properly managed, can have repercussions not only on the quality of care provided to patients, but also on the health and well-being of the caregivers themselves.

The effects of staggered working hours on biological rhythms

Working staggered hours, particularly night shifts or extended on-call duty, disrupts the **circadian rhythm** that regulates our internal clock. This disruption can have immediate effects on sleep, energy and concentration, and longer-term consequences on health.

When the body is forced to function at times when it should normally be at rest, such as at night, it undergoes an **imbalance** that affects sleep, hormones and mood. Daytime sleep, which is often shorter and less restorative than night-time sleep, does not fully compensate for accumulated fatigue. Caregivers, especially those who work alternating days and nights, may find it difficult to fall asleep or to obtain deep, uninterrupted sleep, resulting in chronic fatigue.

Sleep deprivation can also affect **concentration**, decision-making and reflexes, which is of particular concern in the care sector, where every gesture can have significant consequences for patient health. Caregivers working shifted shifts may feel less alert, more prone to making mistakes, or lack patience in the face of difficult situations, amplifying their stress and sense of fatigue.

Physical and emotional fatigue: an exhausting combination

In addition to the fatigue associated with working long hours, caregivers also have to cope with an **intense emotional burden**. Caring for seriously ill patients, accompanying families in their anguish or bereavement, and witnessing suffering on a daily basis all lead to psychological fatigue that accumulates over time.

The **emotional burden** results from constant contact with pain, illness and death. Caregivers are often on the front line, assisting patients at difficult times, sometimes in the terminal phase, or after major operations. This proximity to human suffering, even for trained and seasoned professionals, can lead to what is known as **compassion fatigue**. This phenomenon occurs when caregivers, overly exposed to their patients' suffering, experience an emotional exhaustion that reduces their capacity for empathy and compassion.

What's more, **managing families** and accompanying them at critical moments adds an extra dimension to this emotional burden. The weight of relatives' expectations, fears or sadness is added to the responsibility of providing physical care to patients. This can create a **heightened** sense of **responsibility**, which translates into even greater psychological fatigue. When a patient dies, or deteriorates despite the care provided, some caregivers may feel a sense of **guilt** or **frustration**, even though they know rationally that they have done all they can. These emotions, combined with physical fatigue, can lead to generalized exhaustion.

Impact on the physical and mental health of caregivers

Staggered working hours and emotional strain have deleterious effects on **caregivers' overall health**. On a physical level, chronic sleep deprivation can weaken the immune system, making caregivers more vulnerable to infections, cardiovascular disease, and metabolic disorders such as diabetes. Digestive disorders are also common among night shift workers, due to irregular mealtimes and an often unbalanced diet.

Accumulated fatigue can also lead to problems of **musculoskeletal pain**, particularly among caregivers who perform heavy physical tasks, such as mobilizing patients or providing prolonged bed care. Lack of rest prevents proper muscle recovery, which can aggravate pain and make technical movements more difficult to perform.

On a mental level, unmanaged **emotional fatigue** can lead to **burnout**, a professional exhaustion characterized by a loss of interest in work, reduced performance, and emotional detachment from patients. Burned-out caregivers may experience a constant sense of exhaustion, increased irritability, and difficulty finding meaning in their work, altering their relationship with patients and colleagues. In the most severe cases, this can lead to **anxiety** or depressive **disorders**.

Strategies for managing fatigue and emotional stress

To alleviate the effects of fatigue linked to shifting working hours and emotional load, it is essential to implement **stress management** strategies and maintain a certain balance between professional and personal life.

Managing sleep and work schedules

One of the first levers for better fatigue management is to **adapt to staggered working hours** by adopting rituals that promote quality sleep. This can include simple measures such as using **blackout curtains** to promote sleep during the day, limiting caffeine consumption before rest, or creating a **bedtime routine** that signals the body that it's time to relax, even outside the usual hours.

It is also important to respect **sufficient rest** periods between shifts, and to avoid accumulating too many working hours without adequate breaks. Caregivers must take care to listen to their bodies and ask for support if the workload becomes too heavy.

Emotional support and mutual aid

On an emotional level, **communication within the team** is crucial. Talking about feelings with colleagues, sharing difficulties encountered, and supporting each other helps to lighten the emotional load. Some departments set up **debriefing** sessions after difficult events, such as a death or critical situation, to enable caregivers to express their emotions and release accumulated stress.

Psychological support can also help. Talking to a mental health professional can help put stress and emotional fatigue into words, and identify strategies to better manage work-related emotions. Some facilities offer support programs for caregivers, such as consultations with a psychologist or workshops on stress management.

Taking time for yourself and preserving your personal balance

Finally, it's essential that caregivers take **time for themselves** outside work to preserve their personal equilibrium. Regular physical activity, relaxing outside the hospital environment, and maintaining social ties are all ways to **recharge their batteries** and recover both physically and mentally. Even moderate physical activity helps combat chronic fatigue and improves sleep quality.

Taking time out for yourself, away from your professional responsibilities, helps you **recharge your batteries** and regain the energy you need to face the challenges of the workplace. These moments of relaxation are essential to prevent fatigue from becoming a permanent condition, and to preserve the passion and satisfaction that comes from working with patients.

Chapter 7

Emergency management in gastroenterology

1 Identify and react quickly to critical situations

- Signs of hemorrhagic shock and management of digestive bleeding

Hemorrhagic shock is a medical emergency that occurs when the body suffers severe blood loss, compromising blood circulation and oxygenation of vital organs. In gastroenterology, digestive hemorrhage is a frequent cause of this type of shock, whether acute or chronic. Management of digestive bleeding requires rapid, coordinated attention, involving identification of the signs of hemorrhagic shock, stabilization of the patient, and implementation of measures to stop bleeding and prevent complications.

Signs of hemorrhagic shock: recognizing the emergency

Hemorrhagic shock occurs when the amount of blood circulating in the body decreases significantly, resulting in a reduced supply of oxygen to tissues and organs. It is essential to identify the **clinical signs** early, so that action can be taken before shock becomes irreversible.

Vital signs and clinical manifestations

The first signs of hemorrhagic shock usually include **tachycardia** (increased heart rate) and **hypotension** (reduced blood pressure). The heart speeds up to compensate for blood loss and maintain organ perfusion. As blood volume decreases, blood pressure falls, further compromising tissue oxygenation.

Skin **paleness** is also observed, linked to peripheral vasoconstriction, the body's response to redirect blood to vital organs. The **skin becomes cold and clammy**, a sign that the body is entering a compensation phase to preserve essential organs such as the heart and brain. Other symptoms include **decreased urine output** (oliguria) and **mental confusion**, signs of poor renal and cerebral perfusion.

At a more advanced stage, the patient may experience **breathing difficulties** (polypnoea(, as the body tries to compensate for the drop in oxygenation. **The patient's consciousness** may also deteriorate, moving from initial confusion to drowsiness, or even coma if the shock is not treated quickly.

Specific signs of digestive hemorrhage

In gastroenterology, acute digestive hemorrhage may be revealed by more specific signs, such as **melena** (black, tarry stools) or **hematemesis** (vomiting of blood). Melena is a sign of bleeding in the upper gastrointestinal tract, often associated with gastric or duodenal ulcers, or ruptured esophageal varices.

Hematochezia (bright red blood in the stool) may also be observed, particularly in cases of bleeding from the lower segments of the digestive tract, such as diverticulosis or colonic lesions. These signs should immediately alert the health-care team to the seriousness of the situation and the need for urgent treatment.

Management of gastrointestinal bleeding: stabilizing the patient

The management of digestive bleeding follows a well-defined protocol, aimed at stabilizing the patient, stopping the bleeding and preventing complications. The first steps are to assess the severity of the bleed, restore circulating blood volume, and identify and treat the source of bleeding.

Initial management and stabilization

The **immediate priority** in the event of hemorrhagic shock is to stabilize the patient's hemodynamic state. Placing the patient in a supine position with legs elevated promotes cerebral perfusion. At the same time, one or more large-caliber **venous lines** can be set up to allow rapid administration of resuscitation fluids (crystalloids or colloids) to compensate for the loss of blood volume and restore arterial pressure.

If shock is severe, **blood transfusion** may be rapidly required to restore blood volume and improve tissue oxygenation. Monitoring of vital parameters (blood pressure, heart rate, oxygen saturation) is essential during this phase, as is assessment of digestive blood loss (volume and appearance of blood released).

In parallel, **oxygen** administration is often essential to maximize tissue oxygenation, especially if perfusion is compromised by blood loss. Oxygen saturation and respiratory status are monitored to verify the effectiveness of this measure.

Finding the source of bleeding

Once the patient is stabilized, the next step is to identify the **source of the bleeding**. This is usually done by means of an endoscopic examination, such as **gastroscopy** or **colonoscopy**, depending on the presumed location of the bleeding. These examinations not only identify the source of the bleeding, but also enable us to intervene to stop it.

For example, if a bleeding **ulcer** is detected, endoscopic treatments such as vasoconstrictor injections, thermocoagulation or hemostatic clips may be used to stop the bleeding. In the case of **esophageal varices**, elastic ligation or injection of sclerosing agents is often performed.

If the source of bleeding is inaccessible, or if endoscopy cannot effectively control it, more invasive techniques may be considered, such as **arterial embolization** by interventional radiology, or in some cases, surgical intervention.

Long-term management and prevention of recurrence

Once acute bleeding has been managed, the priority is to prevent recurrence. This involves **treating the underlying causes** and closely monitoring the patient. For example, if the bleeding is due to a peptic ulcer, it is essential to treat the **Helicobacter** pylori infection (where present) and to introduce proton pump inhibitor (PPI) therapy to reduce gastric acidity and promote healing.

In the case of esophageal varices, prophylactic treatments, such as the use of **beta-blockers**, can be introduced to reduce portal pressure and prevent recurrence of bleeding. In addition, regular endoscopic monitoring is often necessary to identify and treat new lesions before they become symptomatic.

It's also important to manage **risk factors** in patients at risk of bleeding recurrence, such as alcoholism or chronic use of non-steroidal anti-inflammatory drugs (NSAIDs), which promote digestive ulceration and bleeding.

- Management of intestinal perforations and other abdominal emergencies

The management of intestinal perforations and abdominal emergencies is one of the most critical situations in gastroenterology. These conditions, whether related to intestinal perforation, appendicitis, occlusion or peritonitis, require rapid and rigorous intervention to avoid serious or even fatal complications. These life-threatening emergencies often require a multidisciplinary team to ensure optimal management, from early recognition of symptoms to surgical or medical management of the emergency.

Intestinal perforations: diagnosis and immediate management

An **intestinal perforation** occurs when a segment of the intestine, whether small or colonic, is breached, allowing digestive contents to escape into the abdominal cavity. This type of emergency is usually caused by severe ulceration (as in Crohn's disease or peptic ulcers), abdominal trauma, intestinal ischemia, or iatrogenic causes (such as perforation after colonoscopy).

The diagnosis of intestinal perforation is based on suggestive clinical signs and further investigations. Patients often present with **acute**, intense, well-localized **abdominal** pain, rapidly accompanied by **abdominal rigidity** ("plastron" abdomen) due to peritonitis, an inflammation of the peritoneum secondary to irritation by bacteria and digestive contents. The patient may also experience **nausea**, **vomiting** and **cessation of transit**.

Diagnostic tests and clinical signs

Clinical signs of intestinal perforation include intense pain and **abdominal contracture**, but also signs of sepsis such as **tachycardia**, **fever** and sometimes a **drop in blood pressure**. This is a condition that can rapidly progress to septic shock if management is delayed.

Diagnosis is confirmed by **imaging tests**, mainly an abdominal X-ray, which can reveal **pneumoperitoneum** (free air under the diaphragm), or a more sensitive **abdominal CT scan**, which can pinpoint the exact location of the perforation and assess the extent of inflammation or infection.

Initial management and stabilization of the patient

Management of an intestinal perforation begins with **stabilizing** the patient. Administration of **intravenous fluids** is crucial to correct dehydration and maintain blood pressure. At the same time, **broad-spectrum antibiotic therapy** is initiated to treat bacterial contamination of the peritoneum and prevent progression to severe peritonitis or septic shock.

Stopped transit and abdominal distension are also managed by placement of a nasogastric **tube** to decompress the stomach and limit vomiting or reflux. **Oxygen therapy** may be required to stabilize respiratory parameters if the patient's hemodynamic state deteriorates.

Surgical procedure

Once the patient is stabilized, **surgery** is generally the treatment of choice to repair the perforation and treat associated peritonitis. Depending on the cause and location of the perforation, surgery may involve **suturing of the breach**, resection of the perforated segment, or **temporary colostomy** to allow discharge of digestive contents and promote healing of the injured area.

In some cases, a **minimally invasive** laparoscopic approach may be considered if conditions allow, but a conventional **laparotomy** is often necessary, especially in cases of generalized peritonitis or multiple abscesses. The decision on surgical approach depends on the extent of peritoneal contamination, the patient's condition, and the underlying cause of perforation.

Other abdominal emergencies: appendicitis, occlusions and peritonitis

In addition to intestinal perforation, several other abdominal emergencies may require prompt attention, including appendicitis, intestinal obstruction and peritonitis.

Acute appendicitis

Acute appendicitis is a frequent surgical emergency, manifesting as localized abdominal pain, usually in the right iliac fossa, accompanied by nausea, moderate fever and tenderness to palpation. If the appendix becomes necrotic or perforated, localized or generalized peritonitis may occur.

Diagnosis is often confirmed by **abdominal CT scan**, although ultrasound is also useful, particularly in children and pregnant women. Treatment consists of **appendectomy**, performed either laparoscopically or by laparotomy in the case of diffuse peritonitis.

Antibiotics are essential in complicated forms, and post-operative monitoring is necessary to avoid complications such as intra-abdominal abscesses or adhesions.

Intestinal occlusions

Intestinal obstruction is another gastrointestinal emergency, manifesting as cessation of transit, vomiting, abdominal pain and distension. It can be caused by post-surgical adhesions, hernias, tumors or volvulus.

Diagnosis is based on clinical examination and imaging studies, in particular abdominal CT scans, to identify the obstruction, its cause and possible complications, such as ischemia or perforation.

Initial management consists **of decompressing the intestine** with a nasogastric tube, rehydrating the patient intravenously, and closely monitoring progress. In the event of **complete** or complicated **obstruction** (intestinal strangulation, ischemia), surgery is required to remove the obstruction, sometimes by resection of the necrotic area.

Acute peritonitis

Acute peritonitis can result from intestinal perforation, complicated appendicitis, or abdominal infection such as cholecystitis or diverticulitis. It manifests as intense abdominal pain, abdominal wall contracture and signs of sepsis, such as fever, tachycardia and hypotension.

Management is based on **rapid resuscitation** with intravenous fluids, administration of broad-spectrum antibiotics, and emergency surgery to treat the underlying cause of peritonitis. Depending on the cause, surgery may involve draining an abscess, repairing a perforation, or resecting a segment of the bowel.

Post-operative care and prevention of complications

After surgical management of an abdominal emergency, post-operative care is crucial to promote a good recovery and prevent complications. Close monitoring of **vital parameters**, surgical wound status and digestive function is essential.

The risk of **post-operative infections** (intra-abdominal abscess, wound infection) must be taken into account, sometimes necessitating prolonged antibiotics or abscess drainage. Resumption of bowel function is also a key factor to be monitored: early resumption of oral feeding, subject to good bowel function, helps to speed recovery.

Long-term complications, such as **adhesions** or **digestive fistulas**, can occur after complex abdominal surgery, especially in cases of severe peritonitis or prolonged occlusions. Regular monitoring and follow-up consultations are necessary to detect these complications early and adjust treatment.

- Management of incoercible vomiting and severe dehydration

The management of incoercible vomiting and severe dehydration is a frequent medical emergency, particularly in gastroenterology, where many pathologies can lead to these symptoms. Incoercible vomiting, which is persistent and difficult to control, can rapidly lead to severe dehydration, electrolyte imbalance, and other serious complications if prompt management is not implemented. A systematic and rigorous approach is essential to stabilize the patient, identify the underlying cause, and institute appropriate treatment to correct fluid losses, while providing relief from vomiting.

Incoercible vomiting: assessment and clinical signs

Incoercible vomiting, by its repetition and persistence, can be associated with a variety of causes, such as gastrointestinal infections, intestinal obstruction, acute gastritis, metabolic diseases, or the side-effects of drugs or treatments such as chemotherapy. In some cases, neurological conditions such as migraine, or hormonal imbalances such as hyperemesis gravidarum (pregnancy-related), may also be responsible.

The challenge in managing uncontrollable vomiting is first to assess the patient's state of severity. When prolonged, vomiting leads to a significant loss of fluids and electrolytes, particularly sodium, potassium and chlorine, rapidly leading to **severe dehydration** and hydroelectrolytic disorders. The loss of hydrochloric acid due to gastric vomiting can also lead to **metabolic alkalosis**, which, if left uncorrected, can worsen the patient's condition.

Clinical signs to watch out for in the event of uncontrollable vomiting include **tachycardia** (rapid heart rate), a **drop in blood pressure**, **dry mucous membranes**, **reduced diuresis**, and **muscle cramps**. General weakness, dizziness and even mental confusion are also signs that should alert you to the seriousness of dehydration.

Severe dehydration: symptoms and complications

Severe dehydration is a medical emergency in its own right, occurring when fluid losses exceed intake. It manifests as intense thirst, dry mouth, sunken eyes and loss of skin elasticity. **Bedridden or elderly patients**, as well as those with co-morbidities, are particularly at risk of severe dehydration, as they often fail to compensate with adequate fluid intake.

In addition to skin and mouth signs, there are more serious signs such as **orthostatic hypotension** (drop in blood pressure when standing), **oliguria** (reduced urine output), **difficulty concentrating**, and even **impaired consciousness**. These symptoms indicate that the perfusion of vital organs has been compromised, with a risk of progression to **hypovolemic shock** if dehydration is not rapidly treated.

Biologically, blood tests may reveal **hypernatremia** (excess sodium), a sign of severe dehydration, and **electrolyte disorders**, such as hypokalemia (low potassium), which can cause cardiac arrhythmias. Blood gases may also indicate **metabolic alkalosis**, particularly in cases of prolonged vomiting.

Initial management of intractable vomiting and dehydration

The management of incoercible vomiting and severe dehydration is based on two main principles: **stabilizing the patient** and **correcting fluid and electrolyte losses**. The therapeutic approach must be rapid and adapted to the patient's clinical condition.

Intravenous rehydration

Intravenous rehydration is the essential first step in the management of incoercible vomiting and dehydration. A large-bore **peripheral venous** line should be inserted to allow rapid administration of rehydration solutions. **Saline** (0.9% NaCl) or **Ringer's lactate** solutions are often used to correct hypovolemia. The amount of fluids administered depends on the patient's state of dehydration, assessed on the basis of clinical signs, patient weight and estimated losses.

In cases of moderate to severe dehydration, intakes of 1 to 3 liters of fluids are generally required within the first few hours. **Vital parameters** (blood pressure, heart rate) and **diuresis** must be monitored to assess response to rehydration.

Correction of electrolyte imbalances

Electrolyte disorders must also be corrected in parallel with rehydration. The administration of **potassium** is crucial, particularly in the case of hypokalemia, which is common with prolonged vomiting. Severe hypokalemia can lead to serious cardiac complications, such as arrhythmias, and must therefore be corrected under close supervision.

Bicarbonate supplementation may also be considered if metabolic alkalosis is severe and compromises the patient's acid-base balance. Electrolytes should be monitored regularly via blood tests to adjust intake to the patient's needs.

Antinauseants and antiemetics

Relief of incoercible vomiting requires the administration of appropriate **antiemetics**, to stop the vomiting cycle and improve patient comfort. Among the most commonly used molecules are **serotonin (5-HT3) receptor antagonists**, such as ondansetron, and **dopamine D2 receptor antagonists**, such as metoclopramide. These drugs act directly on the vomiting centers in the brain, blocking the signals that cause nausea and vomiting.

In certain situations, **antihistamines** or **anticholinergics** may be used, depending on the cause of vomiting (e.g., in cases of vertigo or balance disorders). If vomiting is chemically induced, more specific treatment may be required, sometimes involving **corticosteroids** or NK1 (neurokinin 1) receptor antagonists.

Identifying and treating the underlying cause

While incoercible vomiting and severe dehydration are emergencies that need to be treated quickly, it's just as important to **identify the underlying cause in** order to prevent a recurrence. The etiology of incoercible vomiting can be varied, and each cause requires specific treatment.

In cases of acute **gastrointestinal infection**, it is important to treat the infection itself, sometimes with antibiotics or antiparasitics depending on the infectious agent identified. For patients suffering from **intestinal obstruction, mechanical obstruction** or **ileus**, appropriate surgical or medical management may be required, including placement of a nasogastric **tube** to decompress the stomach and relieve vomiting.

In cases of **acute gastritis** or **peptic ulcers**, the prescription of proton pump inhibitors (PPIs) is essential to reduce gastric acidity and promote healing of lesions. Pregnancy-related vomiting, as in **hyperemesis gravidarum**, requires specific management, with appropriate nutritional and fluid support.

Prevention and long-term care

Once the acute phase has been managed, it is important to consider **preventive** strategies to avoid recurrence of vomiting and dehydration. Proper patient education on the early signs of dehydration, the importance of adequate hydration, and measures to be taken in the event of recurrence are essential.

For some patients suffering from recurrent vomiting (e.g. in **gastroparesis** or **cyclic vomiting syndrome**), **multidisciplinary management** may be required, involving gastroenterologists, dieticians and supportive care specialists, to optimize long-term treatment.

2 Collaboration with the team in emergency management

•   The caregiver's role in calling the emergency team
The caregiver's role in the call to the emergency team is of crucial importance in ensuring rapid and effective management of critical situations. Although not directly in charge of medical decisions, the caregiver plays a fundamental role in the **early detection of signs of deterioration** in patients, and in the **rapid alerting of** the emergency team. Their expertise, proximity to patients and constant vigilance make them a key player in the emergency care chain.

Observation and identification of emergency signs

The nursing auxiliary is at the forefront of patient observation throughout their hospital stay. Thanks to their regular presence and direct contact with them, they are often the first to perceive **signs of deterioration** or subtle changes in the patient's state of health. These may include changes in vital parameters (drop in blood pressure, tachycardia, reduced oxygen saturation), altered consciousness, sudden or unusual pain, respiratory distress, or symptoms of hemorrhage (vomiting blood, blood in stools).

For example, a patient who suddenly becomes confused or drowsy, despite being alert a few hours earlier, may be showing signs of **neurological failure** or hypoxia. Another example might be a patient whose breathing becomes rapid and shallow, indicating **respiratory distress**. In these cases, the caregiver must immediately assess the seriousness of the situation and decide whether to call the emergency team.

Taking the initiative and communicating effectively

When an **acute event** is detected, the caregiver must be proactive and assertive to quickly alert the emergency team. It's essential that they **take the initiative** to initiate the call without waiting for confirmation from other members of the care team, as every minute counts in critical situations.

The process of calling the emergency team must be methodical and precise. This involves not only dialing the internal emergency number or activating the alarm provided, but also **clearly communicating essential information** to emergency professionals. The caregiver must be able to quickly provide key information such as :

- **Patient identity** (name, age, room)
- **Observed symptoms** (respiratory distress, chest pain, loss of consciousness, etc.)
- **Current vital signs** (heart rate, blood pressure, oxygen saturation)
- **Medical background** (patient history, current treatments, last medical assessment)

Clear, concise communication enables the emergency team to arrive on site well informed and ready to intervene immediately.

Preparing the environment before the emergency team arrives

While waiting for the emergency team to arrive, the caregiver must ensure that the **patient is secure** and that the environment is ready to facilitate rapid intervention by the caregivers. This may include simple but crucial gestures, such as :

- **Position the patient correctly**: in the event of respiratory distress, it is important to place the patient in a seated or

215

semi-seated position to facilitate breathing. In the event of syncope or shock, it may be preferable to place the patient in a recumbent position, with legs elevated to promote cerebral perfusion.

- **Make sure the patient is accessible**: clear objects from around the bed, adjust bedding to allow the team to intervene quickly, and disconnect any non-essential devices that may be in the way.

- **Check medical devices**: the caregiver must ensure that the patient's infusion is working properly, that oxygen is available if necessary, and that all monitoring devices are in place.

- **Prepare equipment**: if a specific intervention is required (for example, in the event of an epileptic seizure or heart attack), the caregiver can prepare certain items according to protocols, such as taking out the emergency cart or ensuring the availability of resuscitation equipment.

Collaboration with the emergency team

Once the emergency team has arrived, the nursing auxiliary plays an essential **support** role. Although they are not directly involved in critical medical procedures (such as cardiopulmonary resuscitation or intubation), they are essential for **providing** additional **information** on the patient's progress, and for assisting the medical team according to their needs.

The nursing auxiliary may also be responsible for practical tasks such as **monitoring vital parameters** while the emergency team intervenes, or **providing logistical assistance** (bringing in equipment, preparing medication, etc.). Their role is to facilitate the team's intervention by remaining responsive and offering effective support, while continuing to look after the patient.

The caregiver may also be responsible for **reassuring the patient and family**. When the emergency team intervenes, it can be an anxious time for the patient and family. By remaining calm and explaining what is happening in a straightforward manner, the caregiver plays a fundamental role in reducing anxiety and fostering a more serene climate around the intervention.

Post-procedure follow-up

After the emergency team has intervened, the caregiver continues to play an important role in **monitoring** the patient, watching for any complications or further deterioration in clinical condition. The patient's situation may remain critical in the hours following an emergency intervention, so **extra vigilance** is essential.

In collaboration with the nursing team, the orderly also participates in the **transmission of information** to the relief teams. These transmissions must include a full description of the incident, the interventions that have been carried out, and the actions to be taken to ensure the patient's safety. This is a crucial step in ensuring continuity of care.

The importance of training and practice

To be effective in their role of alerting and managing emergency situations, orderlies need regular training in **first aid**, **cardiopulmonary resuscitation** and the **emergency protocols** in force in the establishment. Theoretical training must be complemented by practical exercises, such as emergency simulations, so that the orderly feels able to react confidently and quickly in stressful situations.

The ability to remain calm, make the right decisions quickly and communicate effectively is often reinforced by this regular training. Rigorous preparation ensures that, in critical moments, the caregiver can play his or her role to the full and ensure smooth, coordinated patient care.

- Coordination with medical and nursing teams during emergency interventions

Coordination with the medical and nursing teams during emergency interventions is an essential component in ensuring fast, effective and safe patient care. In an emergency, every second counts, and smooth collaboration between the different members of the care team is essential to prevent serious complications or save a life. The caregiver, while not responsible for medical decisions, plays a central role in this dynamic, ensuring continuity of supportive care, communicating effectively with the medical and nursing team, and facilitating interventions at every stage.

Recognizing emergency signs and first reporting

The first stage of coordination in an emergency situation often begins with the caregiver, who is frequently the first to identify **signs of deterioration** in a patient. Whether it's a sudden change in vital parameters, respiratory distress, altered state of consciousness or unusual acute pain, the caregiver must be able to **recognize these early signs** and quickly report the emergency to the nursing and medical team.

At such times, it's crucial for the caregiver to use clear, direct channels of communication. He or she needs to know **who to contact** immediately to trigger intervention (nurses, doctors, in-house emergency team), while remaining calm so as not to aggravate the anxiety of the patient or his or her loved ones. By quickly providing **concise, precise information** on the nature of the deterioration (e.g., "sudden drop in blood pressure" or "rapidly falling oxygen saturation"), the caregiver enables the emergency team to intervene with full knowledge of the situation, and to prepare the necessary actions even before arriving at the patient's bedside.

Preparing the environment prior to intervention

While waiting for the nurses and doctors to arrive, the nursing auxiliary plays an active role in **preparing the environment** so that the medical team can intervene effectively. This includes actions such as :

- **Position the patient** correctly according to his or her condition (e.g. in the event of respiratory distress, elevate the chest, or lay the patient down in the event of shock).
- **Prepare the necessary equipment**: check that monitoring equipment (oxygen, infusion, blood pressure monitor) is functional and that the emergency cart is available and ready for use if necessary.
- **Create an environment conducive to the procedure**: clear the area around the patient to facilitate access for caregivers, and ensure that other medical devices (catheters, infusions, etc.) do not interfere with the procedure.

By taking these steps, the caregiver optimizes the intervention environment and enables the emergency team to focus immediately on assessing and stabilizing the patient, without wasting time.

Collaboration and support during intervention

Once the medical and nursing team arrives, the caregiver must hand over the baton while continuing to **play an active support role**. The first step is to provide a **rapid and accurate report** on the patient's condition, indicating what has been observed (symptoms, vital parameters), what actions have been taken, and any other relevant factors (for example, the patient's recent medication or ongoing treatment). This transmission of information is essential if nurses and doctors are to have an overview of the situation and be able to make informed decisions.

While the medical team carries out assessment and medical interventions (resuscitation, intubation, administration of emergency medication), the caregiver continues to play a **logistical support** role. This may include tasks such as:

- **Assist the nurse** by monitoring patient vitals, keeping track of parameters (blood pressure, heart rate, oxygen saturation).
- **Provide equipment**: make sure the medical team has all the necessary equipment (drugs, syringes, resuscitation equipment).
- **Respond to specific requests from caregivers**, whether to provide specific devices or reposition the patient according to the team's needs.

Throughout the intervention, it's crucial for the caregiver to maintain a **calm, proactive** attitude, while remaining attentive to the needs of the emergency team. His or her ability to anticipate the needs of caregivers and respond quickly to requests contributes to a smooth intervention, enabling the medical team to concentrate on stabilizing the patient.

Role in communication and continuity of care

Effective communication between the different members of the care team is essential to ensure **continuity of care** after the emergency intervention. Once the patient is stabilized, the caregiver collaborates with the nurses to **monitor clinical progress** and detect any complications or relapses. This may include monitoring vital parameters, managing medical devices, and administering comfort or supportive care.

The caregiver must also ensure that all important information is passed on to the relief medical team during team changes, or to other professionals who may be involved in the patient's care (resuscitators, surgeons, etc.). This **rigorous transmission** of **information** ensures that every member of the team has a clear and coherent view of the patient's condition and the actions that have been taken.

Managing psychological support for patients and their families

Alongside physical care, the nursing auxiliary plays a fundamental role in providing psychological support for patients and their families during and after an emergency intervention. Emergency situations can be a source of **intense stress** for patients, who may feel frightened or panicked by the medical agitation around them. The caregiver's reassuring approach and straightforward explanations help to ease the patient's anxiety. By adopting a calm, caring attitude, he or she can explain what's going on in an understandable way, without going into technical details that might worry the patient further.

As for **relatives**, who can also be very anxious, the caregiver's job is to inform them of the situation without creating panic. He or she can tell them what the medical team is doing and keep them up to date with the patient's condition, while offering them a space to express any concerns or questions they may have.

• Support for patients and their families at this critical time
Supporting patients and their loved ones at critical moments is a fundamental aspect of healthcare, particularly in emergency situations or at times of great vulnerability. When the patient's prognosis is vital, or their health is deteriorating rapidly, emotional and psychological support becomes just as important as medical management. The caregiver, by virtue of his or her constant proximity to the patient and his or her family, plays a key role in this support. His or her support must be characterized by empathy, benevolence and professionalism, to alleviate anxiety, foster a climate of trust and provide comfort at times when fear and uncertainty dominate.

Emotional support for patients: reassurance and guidance

In critical moments, patients often find themselves immersed in **deep anxiety**, mixed with pain, confusion and vulnerability. Whether the situation is related to a rapidly deteriorating health condition, an emergency intervention or a difficult announcement, the patient may be overwhelmed by intense emotions, including fear of the unknown, of death, or of suffering.

The caregiver plays an essential role in being present and available to the patient. The simple **physical presence** of the caregiver at the patient's side, reassuring eye contact or a gentle word can soothe an anxious patient. At such times, it's important to be **calm and empathetic**, to listen without judgment, and to respond sympathetically to any questions or concerns the patient may express.

Clearly explaining what is happening, in simple, accessible terms, can also help reduce patient anxiety. For example, during an emergency intervention or a complex medical situation, the caregiver can take a few moments to explain the actions taken by the doctors or nurses: "You're going to be given oxygen to help you breathe" or "We're doing everything we can to get you relief quickly". These small explanations help the patient to **regain a degree of control** over the situation, and remove the fear that often stems from incomprehension.

In some cases, the patient may not be able to communicate verbally, due to their state of health (coma, intubation, respiratory distress). At such times, **non-verbal support** becomes even more essential. A comforting gesture, such as holding the patient's hand, adjusting their pillow or simply staying by their side, can provide profound reassurance. This kind of presence, even if silent, sends the patient the message that he is not alone, that he is surrounded and that his suffering is being taken into account.

Supporting loved ones: listening and informing

The presence of loved ones is often a source of comfort for the patient, but it can also be a **source of worry** for them, especially in times of crisis. Seeing a loved one in distress, without being able to help them directly, plunges families into a situation of great emotional vulnerability. Fear of losing a loved one, helplessness in the face of illness, and a lack of understanding of medical procedures can all add to the stress and distress of loved ones.

The caregiver's role at these moments is to **listen actively** and accompany them with empathy. Relatives often need to **understand** what's going on, even if medical or technical terms are not always easy to grasp. It's important to explain clearly the patient's state of health, the care in progress, and what the medical team is planning to do. Sometimes, they are simply looking for reassurance: "Are you doing everything right?" or "How is he doing? The caregiver, although not responsible for medical decisions, can provide soothing answers, without false promises, by remaining transparent yet comforting: "We're doing everything we can to stabilize his condition" or "The medical team is by his side, doing everything they can to make him feel better".

Active listening also means offering loved ones a space to express their **fears, frustrations and concerns**. At such moments, they may feel a multitude of contradictory emotions: anger, sadness, hope, guilt. The caregiver must welcome them with kindness, without judgment, allowing them to verbalize these emotions without immediately seeking to correct them or give them definitive answers.

Managing critical situations: balancing empathy and professionalism

Critical moments require the ability to manage stress, while maintaining a professional attitude. The **caregiver** must strike a

balance between showing empathy to loved ones and the patient, and the **responsiveness** needed to act when the patient's condition worsens or quick decisions need to be made. By remaining calm and structured in their approach, caregivers **help** loved ones feel **supported**, and help prevent panic or anxiety from taking over.

Another important aspect is to **keep** loved ones **regularly informed** of developments, remaining honest and giving them clear updates. They don't always expect immediate solutions, but need to know that the situation is being taken care of, that care is ongoing and that nothing is being left to chance.

In complex medical decisions, or in situations where the prognosis is bleak, families are often faced with difficult choices (for example, when deciding to stop treatment or enter palliative care). At such moments, the caregiver can help by **offering emotional support**: staying present, explaining complex medical terms in a simple, understandable way, and accompanying families through the thought process, without influencing their decisions.

Post-crisis support: continuous presence and follow-up

Once the situation has stabilized, or after a critical event (such as cardiac arrest or emergency surgery), support for the patient and his or her loved ones does not stop. The caregiver must **provide** ongoing **emotional** and psychological **support**. Even after an improvement, patients may still be marked by their experience, with fears about their future and questions about their ability to recover. Post-crisis support can **help the patient rebuild** psychologically, by being available to address his or her concerns and reassuring him or her about future care.

Relatives, for their part, may be emotionally and physically exhausted by the ordeal. Supporting them means continuing to keep them informed of the patient's progress, offering them a space to express their emotions afterwards, and referring them, if necessary, to psychological support services or discussion groups.

3 Managing emotions and stress in emergencies

• Maintaining calm and concentration under pressure
Maintaining composure and focus under pressure is an essential skill, especially in healthcare where emergency situations, patient suffering and relentless demands can create an environment of constant stress. Whether responding to emergencies, managing medical crises or facing critical decisions, the ability to stay in control of one's emotions while remaining focused on priorities is crucial to patient safety and quality of care. This skill is acquired not only through experience, but also through specific strategies and mental preparation adapted to meet the challenges of everyday life in a demanding environment.

The role of calm in stressful situations

Calm is often perceived as a state of mind, but it is above all a **controlled physiological** and emotional response to external stress or pressure. In moments of crisis, such as a sudden deterioration in a patient's condition, panic can set in if caregivers fail to control their emotions. This can not only affect the quality of care, but also increase stress levels for the team and relatives.

Staying calm enables you to **clear your mind**, make more rational decisions and assess priorities in an orderly fashion. For example, when faced with a respiratory emergency, the instinctive reaction might be to act quickly without taking time to reflect. Yet it's in these moments that calm becomes the foundation for making informed choices: checking vital signs, positioning the patient appropriately, calling for help in a structured way. By acting in a calm manner, the caregiver can avoid hasty errors that could compromise the patient's safety.

Concentration under pressure: focus on the essentials

Concentration in a pressurized environment relies on the ability to filter out distractions and focus on **immediate priorities**. Health care, particularly in emergency situations, is often accompanied by a variety of stimuli: noise from machines, conversations, anxiety from loved ones, repeated calls. In this context, it is essential to learn how to **prioritize actions**.

An effective way to maintain concentration is to **mentally structure** the steps to be taken. For example, in the event of cardiac arrest, the caregiver should focus first on the vital steps to be taken: initiating cardiopulmonary resuscitation (CPR), monitoring vital parameters, and delegating certain tasks to other team members. Setting **precise objectives** for each critical moment helps avoid being overwhelmed by the surrounding pressure.

Controlled breathing can be a simple but powerful tool for improving concentration. When under pressure, breathing often becomes shallow and rapid, which can exacerbate stress. Taking deep breaths reduces physiological tension, brings more oxygen to the brain and restores mental clarity.

Manage your emotions to stay on top of your game

Emotions can quickly become overwhelming in life-threatening situations. Fear of doing the wrong thing, anxiety over a tragic event or frustration over a worsening situation can impair the ability to make rational, effective decisions. To maintain calm and concentration, it's crucial to **recognize your emotions** without letting them get the better of you.

One approach is to **take a step back from** the situation, even during moments of crisis. Remembering that each step is a process, that the team is there to collaborate, and that decisions are made gradually, can help put the pressure felt into perspective. For example, in an emergency situation, the caregiver may feel anxious about not intervening quickly enough. However, by concentrating on what they can control (preparing equipment, carefully observing vital parameters, alerting the medical team), they can **transform this anxiety** into concrete, productive action.

It's also important not to **internalize the stress** or emotions of others. Hospital emergency departments are places where suffering, the fear of loved ones and the demands of colleagues can create an atmosphere of collective tension. However, staying focused on one's own responsibilities, without allowing oneself to be overwhelmed by ambient anxiety, helps to maintain a high level of performance.

Anticipation and preparation: the keys to managing pressure

One of the most effective ways of maintaining calm and concentration under pressure is to prepare in advance. **Mental** and technical **preparation** enables you to approach emergency situations with a clear plan, well-established automatisms and the ability to react methodically.

Simulation exercises, frequently used in hospital environments, provide **training for crisis situations** without the real emotional burden. These exercises help reinforce technical skills while training the mind to remain calm in the face of simulated emergencies. When real emergencies arise, these automatisms facilitate stress management, as the actions to be taken are already known and rehearsed.

Anticipating situations also helps **reduce uncertainty**, which is often a source of stress. Knowing where to find emergency tools, mastering intervention protocols, and having a good knowledge of the medical histories of high-risk patients means you can stay focused on the essentials in the event of a crisis.

Communication under pressure: a pillar of concentration

Clear, precise communication is essential to maintain concentration under pressure. In a high-stress environment, the way in which you **communicate with other team members** has a direct influence on the effectiveness of coordination. Speaking concisely, giving precise information about the patient's condition, or formulating clear requests all help to avoid confusion and keep the team aligned on priorities.

Discussions should remain **calm and structured**, even when the situation is critical. Using short sentences, and stating each task explicitly, facilitates decision-making and avoids misunderstandings. For example, in an emergency intervention, saying "I'll check the saturation, please prepare the infusion" clearly directs the actions to be taken and avoids any confusion or wasted time.

Self-care for better pressure management

Maintaining calm and concentration under pressure is not limited to technical or mental skills. The **physical and psychological well-being** of the caregiver is also crucial. Taking care of your body by ensuring a good diet, adequate sleep and regular exercise helps you to better resist stressful situations.

Similarly, **managing stress on a daily basis** through relaxation techniques (such as meditation, cardiac coherence or yoga) helps to improve resilience in the face of professional pressures. These practices help to release accumulated tension and maintain a serene state of mind, even in difficult environments.

- Techniques for managing your own stress and supporting colleagues

Managing your own stress and supporting your colleagues are essential skills in high-pressure professional environments such as the medical field. Caregivers are often exposed to intense situations where urgency, patient suffering and emotional burdens can lead to chronic stress. Knowing how to manage this stress effectively, while offering support to colleagues, is essential to maintaining a healthy working environment, ensuring quality care and preventing burnout. This management relies on both personal strategies and collective actions to create a positive and resilient collaborative dynamic.

Understanding and recognizing your own stress

Before you can effectively manage stress, it's essential to understand its **signs and triggers**. Stress manifests itself differently in different people: some feel physical tension (muscle aches, headaches), others mental agitation (difficulty concentrating, intrusive thoughts), or emotions such as irritability or weariness. Identifying the first signs of stress enables you to deal with them quickly, before they escalate.

The first step is to learn to **listen to your body and mind**. Being aware of the moments when stress rises (for example, before a complex operation, during an emergency situation, or when faced with an overload of work) helps you to adapt your behavior accordingly. This recognition work is fundamental to preventing stress from becoming chronic or spilling over into professional relationships.

Personal stress management techniques

Once stress has been identified, it's essential to adopt techniques to **soothe and manage it** on a daily basis. Among the most effective strategies are **breathing techniques**, which instantly calm the nervous system and refocus the mind. For example, **cardiac coherence** - breathing in for 5 seconds, then out for 5 seconds, for a few minutes - helps to regulate the heartbeat and reduce inner tension.

Conscious breaks are also crucial. In a care environment where caregivers are constantly in demand, it's easy to forget ourselves and never take a step back. Yet short breaks - even just a few minutes - to stretch, have a glass of water, or simply take a deep breath, can **relieve the pressure and** allow you to return to work more focused and serene. These moments shouldn't be seen as a waste of time, but as a necessary **recharge** to maintain performance and avoid overwork.

Priority management is another pillar of stress management. Knowing how to organize your day according to what is really urgent and important helps you to avoid feeling overwhelmed by the tasks at hand. It's useful to create a **task list** and prioritize actions according to their immediate impact on patient care. This helps to maintain a clear vision and avoid being overwhelmed by the sheer volume of work.

Regular physical activity is also essential for relieving accumulated stress. Physical exercise releases endorphins, the feel-good hormones, and reduces muscle tension caused by stress. Whether it's walking, yoga, swimming or jogging, finding an activity that provides physical exercise helps maintain mental equilibrium.

Taking care of yourself to better take care of others

A fundamental aspect of stress management is the idea that a caregiver must first **take care of themselves before** they can offer quality care to others. This means maintaining a **balanced lifestyle**: getting a good night's sleep, eating healthily, and taking time out from work to relax.

Sleep, for example, plays a crucial role in our ability to manage stress. Insufficient or poor-quality sleep can accentuate fatigue, reduce concentration and make you more vulnerable to the pressures of the day. That's why it's essential to maintain a **regular sleep pattern**, even when working shifts. A good sleep routine ensures that you wake up rested and ready to face the challenges of the day.

It's also important to preserve moments of **disconnection**, away from the professional environment. Giving yourself time for yourself, whether through hobbies, creative activities or simply moments of calm, helps you to regenerate mentally. These periods of disconnection enable you to step back from the stresses of work and avoid emotional exhaustion.

Supporting colleagues in managing stress

In an environment as demanding as that of healthcare, support among colleagues is fundamental. Working in a climate of **benevolence and solidarity** creates a framework in which everyone feels supported, even in moments of great pressure. Stress shared by the team can be alleviated when addressed collectively.

Mutual support begins with small daily gestures, such as asking a colleague how they're feeling, offering to help when they're overwhelmed, or simply listening when they need to talk. These simple gestures strengthen the bond between team members and create an atmosphere of **trust and cooperation**.

It's also important to **recognize the signs of stress** in others. Sometimes, a colleague may be overwhelmed without even realizing it, or may not dare ask for help. Spotting the signs of exhaustion (irritability, visible fatigue, isolation) and offering proactive support can defuse situations that could lead to burn-out.

Encouraging **joint breaks**, especially during busy periods, is a way of taking a moment to breathe together, talk things over and release the pressure. These moments of collective pause reinforce team cohesion and remind us that everyone is there to support each other.

Communication as a lever for support

Open, non-judgmental **communication** is the key to supporting colleagues. Expressing one's feelings, sharing experiences and discussing the difficulties encountered not only relieves one's own stress, but also helps others to feel less alone in their difficulties. **Debriefing** moments after difficult interventions or stressful situations are invaluable in enabling everyone to talk about how they felt, and thus reduce the build-up of unexpressed tensions.

It's also important to **avoid judgment or criticism** when a colleague shows signs of fatigue or stress. The aim should be to create an environment where caregivers feel safe to express their vulnerabilities without fear of appearing weak. This involves **active listening**, genuine attention to what the other is expressing, and affirmative verbal support: "You're doing a good job", "Don't hesitate to ask for help if you need it".

Encouraging collective resilience

Collective resilience is the ability of a team to overcome challenges together and emerge stronger. By actively supporting his or her colleagues, the caregiver contributes to the creation of a **culture of mutual support**, where everyone feels responsible for the well-being of the other. This translates into a dynamic where, in the event of a work overload or crisis situation, team members share tasks in a flexible and adaptable way.

A resilient work environment is also built by setting up moments of **collective reflection**, where the team can discuss stress management practices, share tips, and encourage each other to adopt behaviors that promote well-being. These discussions reinforce cohesion and a shared commitment to maintaining good mental and physical health.

Chapter 8

The use of technologies and medical devices in gastroenterology

1 Understanding and handling devices used in gastroenterology

- Enteral and parenteral feeding pumps: operation and monitoring

Enteral and parenteral feeding pumps play an essential role in the management of patients who are unable to take oral nourishment due to digestive disorders, serious illness or surgery. These devices provide nutrition tailored to the patient's specific needs, while reducing the risk of complications linked to undernutrition or inappropriate nutrient administration. Understanding how they work, and the principles of monitoring, is essential to ensure patient safety and well-being.

Enteral feeding: pump principles and operation

Enteral feeding involves administering nutrients directly into the digestive tract via a tube (nasogastric, nasojejunal or gastrostomy). It is preferred when the digestive tract is functional, but the patient is unable to eat normally, whether due to swallowing disorders, digestive diseases or conditions requiring intensive nutritional support.

Operation of enteral feeding pumps

Enteral feeding pumps are devices that deliver nutrients continuously or intermittently via a digestive tract tube. They ensure controlled feeding in terms of flow rate and volume, thus avoiding the risks of **reaspiration** or **digestive overload**.

These pumps work by delivering liquid nutrition prepared in pouches or containers directly through the probe inserted in the patient's stomach or intestine. The pump's flow rate can be adjusted to meet the patient's individual needs, enabling slow, regular administration over an extended period or at specific times of the day.

The advantage of these pumps is that they can be precisely programmed to adapt the rate of administration (usually in milliliters per hour) and to alert in the event of a problem (probe blockage, end of nutrition, malfunction). Caregivers can thus reliably monitor nutritional intake and adjust parameters as the patient's clinical condition evolves.

Monitoring patients on enteral feeding

Monitoring is essential to prevent complications and ensure that feeding is well tolerated. Several aspects need to be monitored:

1. **Monitoring the catheter site**: It's vital to regularly check the condition of the catheter insertion site, particularly in the case of gastrostomies or jejunostomies. Look for signs of irritation or infection (redness, warmth, discharge), and make sure that the tube is properly secured to prevent any pulling or displacement.

2. **Digestive tolerance**: It is important to monitor symptoms that might indicate intolerance to enteral feeding, such as nausea, vomiting, bloating or diarrhea. Regular monitoring of **gastric residue** (by gently aspirating through the tube to measure the amount of contents in the stomach) can also be carried out to assess whether the patient is tolerating the diet well, particularly in the first few days of administration.

3. **Hydration and diuresis**: Although enteral feeding provides fluids, it is essential to ensure that the patient remains adequately hydrated. The caregiver must monitor the condition of the mucous membranes, diuresis and the appearance of signs of dehydration.

4. **Monitoring vital parameters**: Changes in vital parameters, such as tachycardia or hypotension, may indicate a metabolic or infectious complication, requiring prompt attention.

5. **Pump maintenance**: It's important to check that the pump is working properly, that there are no **blockages** in the probe, that the nutrition bags are properly connected and that nutrition is being delivered at the prescribed rate. If the pump emits an alarm, it should be checked immediately to resolve the problem (low battery, bent or incorrectly positioned probe, etc.).

Parenteral nutrition: pump principles and operation

Parenteral nutrition is used when the patient's digestive system is not functional or cannot be used, as in the case of **malabsorption syndromes**, intestinal obstructions or after certain major surgeries. It involves administering nutrients directly into the bloodstream, often via a central route (such as a central venous catheter) or a peripheral route.

Operation of parenteral nutrition pumps

Parenteral nutrition pumps deliver nutritional mixtures of proteins, carbohydrates, lipids, electrolytes and vitamins directly into the bloodstream, ensuring a complete supply of nutrients.

These pumps enable precise control of the quantity and infusion rate of these nutrient solutions. As with enteral feeding, the use of a pump guarantees **regular, safe** administration, with the possibility of adjusting flow rates according to the patient's needs. Parenteral nutrition pumps must also be configured to avoid infusion errors, such as infusing too rapidly, which could lead to dangerous metabolic imbalances (hyperglycemia, lipid overload, etc.).

Monitoring patients on parenteral nutrition

Parenteral nutrition, while life-saving in certain situations, carries a higher risk of **metabolic and infectious complications**, requiring rigorous monitoring.

1. **Infection monitoring**: Patients receiving parenteral nutrition via a central catheter are at risk of serious infections, such as **sepsis**. It is crucial to monitor the patient's temperature, as well as the condition of the catheter insertion site, for early detection of signs of infection (redness, heat, pain). Catheter management must be rigorous: strict hygiene protocols (hand washing, disinfection of access sites) must be observed to minimize the risk of infection.

2. **Monitoring metabolic imbalances**: Parenteral nutrition may induce imbalances, notably hyperglycemia, hypokalemia or hyperlipidemia. Patients should therefore undergo **regular laboratory tests**, notably to monitor blood glucose, electrolytes, and liver and kidney function tests.

3. **Infusion tolerance**: It is essential to monitor the patient's tolerance to the infusion, in particular by ensuring that nutrition is administered without complication (without local swelling or infiltration at the injection site). Any change in the infusion rate may lead to serious complications, such as volume overload or metabolic disorders.

4. **Monitoring vital parameters**: Close monitoring of vital parameters (heart rate, blood pressure, temperature) is crucial to detect any signs of complications, such as infectious reactions or metabolic destabilization.

5. **Pump operation and maintenance**: The parenteral pump should be checked regularly to ensure that it is operating correctly, that the infusion lines are clear and that the prescribed flow rate is being maintained. Any anomalies or alarms should be immediately checked and corrected.

- Nasogastric tubes and gastrostomy tubes: placement and maintenance

Nasogastric tubes and gastrostomy tubes are essential devices used to administer nutrients, medication or drain fluid when oral feeding is not possible. Their role is particularly crucial in the management of patients suffering from swallowing disorders, chronic diseases affecting the digestive system, or following certain surgical procedures. Although their principle of use is similar, these probes differ in the way they are placed and the length of time they are used. Understanding their operation, placement techniques and maintenance requirements is fundamental to ensuring patient safety and well-being, while reducing the risk of complications.

Nasogastric tubes: placement and maintenance

The nasogastric tube (NGT) is a flexible tube inserted through the nose into the stomach to administer food or medication, or to aspirate gastric contents. This tube is often used in temporary situations, such as enteral feeding or gastric drainage, following surgery, digestive paralysis or gastric decompression.

Nasogastric tube placement

Placing a nasogastric tube is a delicate procedure that must be carried out with great care to avoid complications such as nasal lesions, esophageal irritation or malpositioning in the airway. Before insertion, it is important to explain the procedure to the patient to reduce anxiety and ensure cooperation.

1. **Preparation**: The caregiver or nurse begins by **measuring** the required length of the probe by placing it along the patient's face, from nostril to ear, then down to the base of the sternum. This measurement helps to estimate the

240

insertion depth to ensure that the probe will reach the stomach.

2. **Insertion**: After lubricating the probe to facilitate its passage, insertion is performed through one of the nostrils. The patient is encouraged to swallow during insertion to help the probe progress into the esophagus. It is essential to watch for signs of respiratory discomfort (coughing, choking), which could indicate that the probe is poorly positioned in the airway.

3. **Checking position**: Once the probe is in place, **it** is essential to **check its position** in the stomach before use. The most common method is to **aspirate the gastric contents** to check that the liquid sampled is acidic (pH below 5.5). The other, safer method is to perform an **X-ray** to confirm the location in the stomach, especially when the probe is being placed for the first time or in case of doubt.

Nasogastric tube maintenance

Regular maintenance of the nasogastric tube is essential to avoid obstructions and infections, and to ensure good tolerance.

1. **Nasal site monitoring**: It is important to regularly monitor the **insertion site** for irritation or ulceration of the nostril. Continuous rubbing of the probe can lead to skin lesions and local infections. The probe must be well secured to avoid excessive movement, and nasal care (application of moisturizing creams) may be recommended to limit irritation.

2. **Maintaining catheter patency**: It's crucial to flush the catheter regularly with sterile water or saline solution to avoid **blockages**. This is particularly important after administering medication or thick food. In the event of

blockage, gentle suction or the use of enzymatic products can help unblock the probe.

3. **Monitoring for complications**: It is essential to watch for signs of intolerance to enteral feeding, such as **nausea, vomiting, bloating** or abdominal pain. The patient should also be monitored for signs of a **false route**, particularly in at-risk patients, which could indicate that the tube has moved into the airway.

4. **Removing the tube**: The nasogastric tube can be removed once normal nutrition has been restored, or if it is no longer required. Removal should be carried out with care, after disconnecting any feed or suction, and always taking care not to cause nasal or esophageal lesions.

Gastrostomy tube: placement and maintenance

The gastrostomy tube is a more permanent feeding device than the SNG, inserted directly into the stomach through the abdominal wall. It is used in patients requiring prolonged enteral feeding (several weeks to several months), such as those suffering from severe neurological diseases or head and neck cancers, preventing swallowing.

Gastrostomy tube placement

Placement of a gastrostomy tube is usually performed endoscopically (percutaneous endoscopic gastrostomy or **PEG**) or sometimes surgically. The procedure is performed under local or general anesthesia, depending on the patient's condition.

1. **Endoscopy**: An **endoscope** is inserted through the patient's mouth into the stomach to visualize the interior and guide probe insertion. A small incision is made in the abdominal wall, and the probe is inserted through this opening, directly into the stomach.

2. **Fixing the probe**: Once inserted, the probe is **fixed** inside the stomach with a plate or balloon, while on the outside, a fixation disk holds the probe in place on the skin.

Gastrostomy tube maintenance

Maintaining a gastrostomy tube is essential to avoid local infections, tube displacement or obstructions.

1. **Insertion site care**: The insertion site should be cleaned regularly with saline or sterile water to avoid infection. It is crucial to monitor the area around the probe for signs of irritation, inflammation or gastric **leakage**. In the event of redness, pain or oozing, infection should be suspected and treated promptly.

2. **Preventing blockages**: As with nasogastric tubes, gastrostomy tubes should be rinsed regularly with sterile water after each use, to avoid blockages. It is also advisable to check regularly that the tube is correctly positioned, and that it is not kinked or obstructed.

3. **Monitoring for complications**: It's important to watch for signs of **gastric leakage**, infection of the insertion site or obstruction of the tube. If the tube becomes dislodged, professional reinsertion is often necessary to avoid complications. In addition, nausea, abdominal pain or signs of malabsorption should be monitored to adjust enteral feeding accordingly.

4. **Changing the tube**: The gastrostomy tube must be changed periodically, generally every 6 to 12 months, depending on the type of device. This change is carried out by a healthcare professional under rigorous aseptic conditions to avoid infection.

- Monitoring devices (pulse oximeters, blood pressure monitors)

Monitoring devices, such as pulse oximeters and blood pressure gauges, play a crucial role in tracking patient health, providing vital information on a continuous or intermittent basis. Their use is particularly widespread in intensive care units, emergency departments, and at the bedside of patients whose condition requires close monitoring. These devices enable real-time assessment of cardiovascular and respiratory functions, facilitating early detection of complications and guiding medical decisions. A thorough understanding of their operation, interpretation and maintenance is essential to ensure safe and effective care.

Pulse oximeter: operation and monitoring

The pulse oximeter, also known as a saturometer, is a device that measures **oxygen saturation** in the blood, i.e. the percentage of oxygenated hemoglobin. It also provides a **heart rate** reading. This device is widely used in the monitoring of patients suffering from respiratory or cardiac pathologies, or during surgery, to evaluate in real time the blood's capacity to transport oxygen to the tissues.

Pulse oximeter operation

The pulse oximeter works by means of a probe, usually placed on a finger, toe or earlobe. The device uses **light absorption** technology to measure oxygen saturation. Two beams of light (red and infrared) pass through the tissue, and the amount of light absorbed by oxygenated and deoxygenated hemoglobin is analyzed. The percentage of oxygen saturation is calculated by comparing these two types of absorption. Normal saturation is generally between 95% and 100%, while saturation below 90% indicates **hypoxemia**, requiring intervention.

Pulse oximeter monitoring

Pulse oximeter monitoring is a rapid, non-invasive means of **detecting hypoxia** or respiratory deterioration. It is particularly useful in emergency situations, post-operatively, or during acute respiratory infections such as pneumonia or COPD exacerbations.

1. **Interpretation of values**: It's important to know the normal oxygen saturation value for each patient, as it can vary according to medical history, as in chronic lung disease. A rapid drop in saturation should alert the caregiver to a potential **respiratory compromise**, requiring oxygen administration, rapid medical intervention or reassessment of ventilation.

2. **Patient tolerance and adjustments** : Certain conditions, such as poor peripheral perfusion (due to cold, hypotension or shock), can affect the reliability of oximeter readings. In such cases, probe placement can be adjusted to obtain more accurate values (on a different part of the body), or another device can be used to confirm results.

3. **Alarms and continuous monitoring**: The pulse oximeter can be programmed to sound alarms in the event of low saturation or abnormal heart rate. This feature is essential for patients in intensive care or those on mechanical ventilation, where a rapid drop in saturation could indicate **respiratory distress**.

Tensiometers: operation and monitoring

A blood pressure monitor is a device used to measure **blood pressure**, a key indicator of cardiovascular health. Blood pressure reflects the force exerted by blood against the artery walls, and is generally measured in millimeters of mercury (mmHg). Two values are recorded: **systolic** pressure (when the heart contracts) and **diastolic** pressure (when the heart relaxes between beats).

How tensiometers work

There are two commonly used types of tensiometer: **manual** and **automatic**.

1. **Manual sphygmomanometer**: This type of device requires the use of an inflatable cuff, a stethoscope and a manometer. The cuff is placed around the patient's arm and inflated to compress the brachial artery. Listening to arterial sounds with the stethoscope, the caregiver gradually deflates the cuff, and the first noises heard correspond to **systolic pressure**. When the noises stop, this indicates **diastolic pressure**.

2. **Automatic sphygmomanometer**: More commonly used, it works in a similar way, but does not require a stethoscope. The device automatically inflates the cuff and uses a sensor to detect arterial oscillations, providing a quick and accurate blood pressure reading. These devices are often programmed to monitor blood pressure at regular intervals, making them particularly useful for continuous patient monitoring.

Monitoring with tensiometers

Regular measurement of blood pressure enables us to monitor the patient's hemodynamic status and detect **anomalies** that may indicate clinical deterioration.

1. **Interpretation of values**: Normal blood pressure is around 120/80 mmHg. **Hypotension** (low blood pressure) may indicate shock, severe dehydration or heart problems, while **hypertension** (high blood pressure) may indicate an increased risk of stroke, heart attack or heart failure.

246

Values should be interpreted in the light of the patient's general condition and medical history.

2. **Frequency of measurement**: Depending on clinical condition, blood pressure may be measured at regular intervals (e.g. hourly in intensive care patients), or more frequently in stable patients. In critical cases, continuous monitoring with an **automated blood pressure monitor** is often necessary to follow rapid fluctuations in blood pressure.

3. **Cuff adjustment**: It's important to ensure that the **cuff** is the right size and correctly positioned for an accurate measurement. A cuff that is too large or too small may result in incorrect readings. The cuff should be positioned above the elbow, with the sensor centered on the brachial artery.

Monitoring patients with oximeters and blood pressure monitors

Pulse oximeters and blood pressure monitors provide real-time data to help assess the hemodynamic and respiratory status of patients. Continuous or frequent monitoring with these devices can detect abnormalities before they become serious, which is particularly important in critical care patients.

1. **Early detection of complications**: A drop in oxygen saturation, associated with hypotension, may indicate **shock** or multi-organ failure. Conversely, severe hypertension accompanied by an elevated heart rate may signal **hemodynamic stress** or an inappropriate response to treatment.

2. **Therapeutic adjustments**: Based on measured values, caregivers can adjust oxygen administration, fluid infusion or antihypertensive medication, ensuring that treatment remains adapted to the patient's clinical evolution.

3. **Communication and documentation**: It is essential to accurately **document** all measurements, and to communicate significant changes to members of the medical team. A rapid drop in oxygen saturation, for example, must be reported immediately, as it may require urgent interventions (intubation, assisted ventilation).

Maintenance and proper use of equipment

To guarantee their reliability, monitoring devices must be properly maintained.

1. **Cleaning probes and cuffs**: Pulse oximeters and blood pressure monitors are in direct contact with patients' skin. **Regular disinfection of** probes and cuffs is therefore crucial to avoid cross-contamination.

2. **Calibration check**: Devices must be regularly calibrated to ensure accurate measurements. If a device appears to be giving inconsistent or abnormal readings, even in a stable patient, it should be checked or replaced.

3. **Alarm monitoring**: Caregivers should ensure that oximeter and blood pressure alarms are **activated and set to** appropriate thresholds for each patient, so that any abnormalities are detected immediately.

2 Telemedicine and its impact on gastroenterology

- The contribution of telemedicine to monitoring patients at home

Telemedicine has revolutionized the way patients are monitored and cared for, particularly at home. Thanks to technological advances, it enables care to be extended beyond hospital walls, offering personalized medical follow-up while improving patients' quality of life. This approach is particularly beneficial for people with chronic illnesses, patients in convalescence or those living in remote geographical areas. By facilitating communication between patients and healthcare professionals, telemedicine reduces unnecessary travel, optimizes medical interventions and promotes better pathology management.

Easier access to care and continuity of medical follow-up

One of the major benefits of telemedicine is that it **facilitates access to care**. Patients, especially those who have difficulty travelling, can now benefit from medical follow-up without leaving their homes. For the elderly, or patients with chronic conditions such as heart failure, diabetes or lung disease, this represents a considerable advantage. They can receive regular consultations without having to visit a doctor's surgery, which eases their daily routine and limits the risk of their condition worsening due to tiring or inaccessible travel.

Telemedicine also ensures optimum **continuity of care**, particularly during critical periods. For example, after hospitalization, patients can continue to be monitored regularly via video consultations, thus avoiding repeated or unnecessary hospitalizations. This remote monitoring enables early detection of signs of relapse or complications, facilitating early treatment. Patients are better supervised, while remaining in the comfort of their own home.

Remote surveillance and monitoring of vital parameters

One of the key aspects of telemedicine is **remote** patient **monitoring**, which enables healthcare professionals to monitor crucial vital parameters such as blood pressure, blood sugar, heart rate and oxygen saturation in real time. Using connected devices (oximeters, blood pressure monitors, glucometers, etc.), data is automatically transmitted to the doctor or nurse, without the patient having to go anywhere.

This real-time monitoring enables caregivers to quickly identify **anomalies** or **deteriorations in health status**, such as an abnormal rise in blood sugar levels or a drop in oxygen saturation. This leads to earlier intervention, often before symptoms worsen to the point of requiring hospitalization. Patients with chronic conditions such as hypertension or heart failure benefit from more rigorous monitoring, which can prevent serious complications such as heart attacks or strokes.

Remote monitoring also improves **treatment management**. For example, a diabetic patient can have his or her treatment quickly adjusted in line with observed blood glucose results, without having to wait for the next office consultation. This enables more precise and responsive management of chronic diseases.

Better involvement of patients in their care

Telemedicine encourages greater **patient autonomy** and involvement in managing their health. Thanks to digital tools, patients often have access to their health data in real time, helping them to understand the impact of their treatment and to adapt their daily behavior, particularly with regard to their diet, physical activity or symptom management.

This empowerment is particularly beneficial in the management of **chronic diseases**, where the patient plays an active role. For example, a patient suffering from high blood pressure can monitor his or her blood pressure on a daily basis using a connected blood pressure monitor, and adjust his or her lifestyle according to the results observed. What's more, he can share this information with his doctor via a telemedicine platform, enabling precise adaptation of his treatment.

The involvement of patients in their own care, facilitated by telemedicine, also reinforces **therapeutic compliance**. Regular video consultations and instant feedback from caregivers help keep patients motivated to follow their treatment, respect medical recommendations and adopt healthy lifestyle habits. The patient feels more involved in his or her own health, which in turn boosts adherence to treatment and improves long-term results.

Reduced hospitalization and complications

Another major advantage of telemedicine in monitoring patients at home is the **reduction in hospital admissions** and emergency room visits. Remote monitoring enables early detection of signs of clinical deterioration, which can prevent unnecessary hospitalization or prolonged stays. In heart failure, for example, monitoring blood pressure and heart rate can detect worsening before the situation becomes critical. A simple adaptation of treatment at a distance can then avoid hospitalization.

Telemonitoring also helps prevent **serious complications**, particularly in vulnerable or immunocompromised patients. By reducing travel to hospital environments or doctors' surgeries, telemedicine minimizes the risk of exposure to nosocomial or community-acquired infections, which is particularly important in times of pandemics such as COVID-19. What's more, patients can benefit from remote medical consultations without delaying care due to geographical inaccessibility or mobility problems.

Improving the caregiver-patient relationship

Contrary to popular belief, telemedicine does not isolate patients, but can actually strengthen the **relationship between them and their doctor** or healthcare team. Regular video consultations or exchanges via secure platforms enable **more frequent contact**, without the need to schedule physical consultations. This creates a more fluid relationship, in which the patient feels continuously supported.

Telemedicine also offers caregivers a better understanding of the patient's home environment. During video consultations, the doctor can observe the patient's living environment, identify factors that could influence his or her health (living conditions, stress, organization of home care), and offer appropriate advice.

Equity and accessibility of care

Telemedicine also helps to improve **access to** healthcare for populations that are often deprived of it. Patients living in rural or isolated areas, where access to specialists is limited, can consult doctors remotely, without having to travel long distances. Similarly, people with reduced mobility, or those suffering from serious illnesses, can benefit from regular care without leaving home, avoiding the fatigue and risks associated with travel.

Last but not least, telemedicine helps to overcome **inequalities in access** to certain medical specialties. For example, consultations in dermatology, psychiatry or endocrinology, which can be difficult to access in certain regions, can be carried out via telemedicine platforms, thus reducing waiting times.

- The caregiver's role in remote monitoring of vital parameters

The caregiver's role in remote monitoring of vital parameters is becoming increasingly important with the rise of telemedicine and connected healthcare technologies. Although often associated with local care, the caregiver also plays an essential role in remote monitoring, collaborating with other members of the medical team to ensure **continuous, safe patient care**, while optimizing the quality of care at home. Thanks to their monitoring and care skills, the nursing auxiliary transmits and interprets vital data, while remaining an indispensable link between the patient and the nursing team.

Remote monitoring of vital parameters: a key role in telemedicine

In telemedicine, remote monitoring of vital parameters relies on the use of connected medical devices, such as **pulse oximeters, blood pressure monitors, glucose meters** and **medical scales**. These devices enable real-time monitoring of key patient health indicators such as heart rate, blood pressure, blood glucose, oxygen saturation and body weight.

The caregiver's role is to **support the patient in the use of these** devices, to ensure that they are working properly, and to monitor the results obtained. He/she also acts as a **relay** between the patient and the medical team, rapidly informing healthcare professionals of any anomalies or signs of deterioration in the patient's state of health.

Supporting patients in using remote monitoring devices

One of the caregiver's primary roles is to **train and support the patient** in the use of remote monitoring devices. Many patients, particularly the elderly or those suffering from chronic illnesses, may find it difficult to use these devices independently. The caregiver therefore plays a pedagogical role by explaining how **the devices work**, helping to set up monitoring, and ensuring that measurements are taken correctly and regularly.

For example, for a patient suffering from chronic respiratory insufficiency, the caregiver may show how to use a **pulse oximeter**, explain the frequency of measurements to be taken and indicate normal oxygen saturation values. He or she ensures that the patient is able to monitor his or her parameters independently, but also intervenes to check results or help with technical difficulties.

Data collection and interpretation

Another essential aspect of the caregiver's role is the **collection and monitoring of data** gathered by telemedicine devices. Although the devices are designed to automatically transmit data to medical monitoring platforms, the caregiver remains a key player in the **first-level interpretation of** results and the detection of anomalies.

During home visits or remote exchanges, the caregiver can consult parameters such as blood pressure, weight or blood sugar levels, and **quickly detect deviations** from normal or expected values. For example, in a diabetic patient, a sudden rise in blood sugar levels may indicate an imbalance in treatment or decompensation. The caregiver is then in a position to alert the nursing team for rapid intervention.

This rigorous monitoring helps identify early signs of deterioration, such as hypotension, hyperglycemia or desaturation, which can prevent serious complications and avoid unnecessary hospitalization.

Communication with the care team

Information transmission is one of the caregivers' key functions in remote monitoring. The vital data collected is often analyzed by doctors or nurse coordinators, but it is the caregiver who takes over directly in the event of a critical situation or a worrying change in the patient's condition.

Thanks to their role as **interface** between the patient and the medical team, caregivers can alert healthcare professionals in real time if monitoring results show any anomalies. He or she is also responsible for **transmitting a detailed report** during home visits or interactions with the patient, incorporating not only the parameters measured, but also the overall assessment of the patient's condition (fatigue, clinical signs observed, changes in daily habits).

Working in close collaboration with nurses, doctors and other healthcare professionals, the nursing auxiliary participates in **collaborative care**, enabling treatments to be adapted rapidly or hospitalization initiated if necessary.

Ensuring a relationship of trust and reassurance for the patient

Beyond the technical aspects, the caregiver plays a fundamental role in providing psychological and emotional support to the patient. For many patients, remote monitoring can be a source of anxiety, especially in the absence of regular physical contact with the medical team. The caregiver then becomes a **trusted point of reference**, reassuring the patient of the reliability of remote monitoring and the responsiveness of the care team in the event of a problem.

By remaining available and ready to listen, the caregiver helps to **reinforce the patient's confidence** in the telemedicine system, enabling him or her to feel cared for, even at a distance. This helps to improve patient adherence to care, by involving them more fully in the management of their own health. For example, a hypertensive patient may feel more serene in the knowledge that he or she is being closely monitored, and that his or her blood pressure measurements are constantly reviewed by a professional, even if he or she does not see his or her doctor on a daily basis.

Preventing complications and adjusting care

By regularly monitoring vital parameters and alerting the medical team to any abnormalities, the caregiver plays a crucial role in **preventing complications**. When an anomaly is detected early, it enables **rapid intervention** and adaptation of treatments before the situation worsens. For example, a progressive drop in oxygen saturation in a COPD patient can be treated in time by increasing oxygen therapy, thus avoiding hospitalization for acute respiratory failure.

The caregiver can also intervene to **adjust daily care**, such as encouraging a healthier lifestyle, adapting comfort care, or reminding patients of the importance of adhering to their treatment. This helps optimize the management of chronic illnesses, while reducing the risk of decompensation.

Managing the technical aspects of remote monitoring systems

In addition to their role in monitoring vital parameters, caregivers must also be able to **manage the technical aspects** of using connected medical devices. This includes regularly checking that devices are working properly, resolving minor problems (replacing batteries, adjusting sensors), and assisting patients in the event of technical difficulties.

This technical support is essential to ensure **optimum continuity of monitoring**, without interruptions due to malfunctions. By providing rapid solutions and training patients to use the equipment, the caregiver ensures quality monitoring and minimizes interruptions to vital data collection.

3 Technological innovations in gastroenterology

- Introduction to the endoscopic capsule: a booming technology

The **endoscopic capsule** is a fast-growing technology that is revolutionizing the way doctors explore the digestive tract, particularly the small intestine, an area that remains difficult to access using traditional endoscopic methods. This advance enables parts of the gastrointestinal tract to be viewed and assessed non-invasively, offering a less intrusive and more comfortable alternative to conventional endoscopic techniques such as colonoscopy or gastroscopy.

Introduced in the 2000s, the endoscopic capsule has rapidly established itself as an invaluable tool in the **diagnosis of gastrointestinal pathologies** such as bleeding of obscure origin, inflammatory bowel diseases (such as Crohn's disease), intestinal polyps and tumors. This innovation has expanded the possibilities for investigating the digestive tract, while improving patient comfort and safety.

Endoscopic capsule operating principle

The endoscopic capsule is a capsule-sized device, generally measuring around 11 mm in diameter and 26 mm in length. It is equipped with a small camera, a wireless transmitter, a battery, and sometimes light sources to illuminate the inside of the intestine. The patient ingests the capsule, which travels through the digestive tract throughout the day, transmitting images to an external receiver worn by the patient.

This receiver records thousands of high-resolution images as the capsule progresses through the digestive tract, providing a detailed video of the intestinal mucosa. After completing its journey, the capsule is naturally evacuated in the stool, with no need for retrieval. The recorded data is then transferred to a computer, where it is analyzed by the gastroenterologist for anomalies or signs of pathology.

One of the main advantages of the endoscopic capsule is its ability to explore **the small intestine**, an area often difficult to reach with conventional endoscopic methods. The small intestine, which is several meters long, is not accessible by either upper endoscopy (which explores the esophagus, stomach and duodenum) or colonoscopy (which reaches the colon). Thanks to the capsule, it is now possible to visualize this area, which is crucial for diagnosing certain diseases such as gastrointestinal bleeding of undetermined origin or Crohn's disease.

Endoscopic capsule indications

The endoscopic capsule is used to **assess various pathologies** of the digestive tract, particularly when a more comprehensive exploration is required than that offered by traditional endoscopies. Main indications include :

1. **Search for digestive bleeding**: When a patient shows signs of gastrointestinal bleeding (anaemia, blood in the stool) and conventional examinations fail to identify the source, the capsule can be used to locate active bleeding or responsible lesions in the small intestine.

2. **Diagnosis of Crohn's disease**: The capsule is particularly useful for exploring segments of the small intestine affected by Crohn's disease, especially when the disease is limited to this part and not visible during colonoscopy. It can be used to visualize ulcerations or inflammations characteristic of the disease.

3. **Detecting polyps or tumors**: Although less common than for the colon, monitoring the small intestine can sometimes reveal the presence of **polyps** or **tumors** in this hard-to-reach area. The endoscopic capsule is therefore a valuable tool for detecting these anomalies.

4. **Monitoring celiac disease**: In patients with **celiac disease**, the capsule can be used to assess damage to the intestinal mucosa and monitor treatment efficacy.

Advantages and disadvantages of the endoscopic capsule

The endoscopic capsule offers several **major advantages** over traditional endoscopic techniques. Firstly, it is **minimally invasive**, requiring neither sedation nor extensive medical intervention for insertion. Patients can ingest the capsule independently, and the examination process interferes very little with their daily activities. This contrasts with colonoscopy or gastroscopy procedures, which generally require longer preparation and recovery times, due to the use of sedatives or invasive devices.

Secondly, the capsule enables **complete exploration of the small intestine**, an area often inaccessible to conventional methods. It also provides **high-resolution images** for accurate detection of abnormalities, while reducing the risks associated with invasive procedures such as perforation or infection.

However, the endoscopic capsule also has a number of **limitations**. Unlike traditional endoscopies, it cannot be used for biopsies or therapeutic interventions. If a suspicious lesion is discovered, endoscopy or surgery may be required to confirm the diagnosis or treat the pathology. What's more, in some patients, particularly those suffering from intestinal **stenosis** (narrowing of the digestive tract), the capsule could become blocked, leading to complications. For this reason, prior tests are often carried out to assess the risk of obstruction before using the capsule.

Finally, although the technology is expanding rapidly, its cost remains relatively high, which may limit its accessibility in certain regions or for certain patients.

Perspectives and innovations

The scope of the endoscopic capsule is constantly evolving, and numerous innovations are underway to further enhance its diagnostic capabilities. For example, new-generation capsules include **magnetic navigation** systems, enabling better control of the capsule inside the body for more targeted exploration.

Research is also underway to develop capsules capable of **taking biopsies** or performing **minimally invasive procedures**, which would considerably increase their therapeutic potential. In addition, the integration of **artificial intelligence** in the analysis of images captured by the capsule would facilitate the detection of anomalies and improve diagnostic accuracy.

- New remote monitoring and diagnosis techniques

New remote monitoring and diagnosis techniques are profoundly transforming the healthcare landscape. Thanks to the rapid evolution of digital technologies, it is now possible to monitor patients' health, make early diagnoses and track the progress of illnesses without the need for a physical visit to a doctor's surgery or hospital. These innovations enable a more proactive approach to care, improving the management of chronic diseases, the prevention of complications and access to care for remote or vulnerable populations. These advances, grouped together under the general term of **telemedicine**, cover a wide range of tools and connected devices that are redefining the relationship between caregivers and patients.

Remote monitoring and follow-up systems

One of the most revolutionary aspects of new remote monitoring techniques is the use of **connected medical devices** to **monitor vital parameters** and other health indicators. These devices enable caregivers to monitor crucial data such as heart rate, blood pressure, blood sugar and oxygen saturation in real time, without the patient having to leave home.

Connected oximeters, blood pressure monitors and glucometers

Connected pulse oximeters, **blood pressure monitors** and **glucose meters** are common examples of these technologies. These devices are equipped with sensors that automatically collect data and transmit it to secure platforms where it can be analyzed by healthcare professionals. This enables **continuous monitoring** of patients with chronic conditions such as heart failure, diabetes or high blood pressure. For example, for a diabetic patient, a connected glucometer can monitor blood sugar levels in real time, enabling treatment to be adjusted more reactively. Similarly, a COPD patient can be equipped with a connected oximeter that alerts the care team to any dangerous drop in oxygen saturation.

These devices help **prevent hospitalization** by detecting signs of deterioration well before the onset of serious symptoms. In this way, they offer **preventive management** that improves patient outcomes while reducing healthcare costs.

Connected medical scales and motion sensors

Connected medical scales, often used to monitor heart failure patients, enable early detection of fluid retention linked to worsening disease. Weight is an indirect indicator of cardiac health, and any significant variation may require treatment adjustment. Combined with other devices, such as **motion sensors**, these scales offer a global view of the patient's state of health, making it possible to monitor not only vital signs, but also physical activity, an important indicator for patients undergoing rehabilitation or at risk of falling.

Connected watches and bracelets

More and more patients are also using **connected watches or bracelets** that continuously measure data such as heart rate, physical activity level, sleep quality, and even electrocardiogram (ECG). These devices can alert both patient and caregiver to anomalies, such as a heart rhythm disorder or an episode of tachycardia. This technology enables **proactive detection of** health problems, even before serious symptoms appear, which is particularly useful for patients at risk of cardiovascular accidents.

Teleconsultation and remote medical monitoring

Teleconsultation has become one of the pillars of remote care, especially since the COVID-19 pandemic accelerated its widespread adoption. Teleconsultation enables patients to **consult their doctor remotely**, via a secure platform, without having to travel. This is particularly advantageous for the elderly, patients living in rural areas, or those whose state of health does not easily allow them to visit a physical consultation.

This type of monitoring is particularly useful for the management of **chronic diseases**, where patients can benefit from regular consultations with their GP or a specialist, to adjust their treatment or discuss the evolution of their pathology. Thanks to **real-time data transmission** from connected devices, the doctor has a precise view of the patient's state of health at the time of consultation.

At the same time, **tele-expertise** platforms enable healthcare professionals to seek specialist advice remotely for complex cases, facilitating **medical collaboration** and reducing waiting times for certain diagnoses.

Artificial intelligence and predictive analysis

Artificial intelligence (AI) technologies add an extra dimension to remote monitoring and diagnosis. By integrating AI algorithms into telemonitoring platforms, it becomes possible to analyze collected health data in real time, and identify **trends or anomalies** that the human eye might not immediately detect. For example, AI can be used to analyze **telemedicine data** and predict a worsening in a patient's state of health before it is clinically visible.

A concrete example of this application is the analysis of **remote ECG data**. By combining data from multiple patients, AI can learn to detect cardiac arrhythmias with greater accuracy, enabling faster intervention. Similarly, in monitoring chronic diseases such as diabetes, AI systems can help adjust insulin doses based on blood glucose trends detected over several days.

Capsules and remote diagnostic devices

Recent innovations include devices capable **of remote diagnosis**, such as **endoscopic capsules**. These small capsules, ingested by the patient, contain a miniature camera that captures images of the inside of the gastrointestinal tract. These images are then transmitted remotely to the medical team to assess the condition of the intestinal mucosa, looking for signs of bleeding, inflammation or polyps. This type of technology makes it possible to carry out in-depth examinations without the patient having to undergo an invasive procedure or go to hospital.

Innovations such as **connected patches** or **skin sensors** also enable continuous physiological data (such as body temperature, electrical activity of the heart or perspiration levels) to be collected and transmitted remotely. These discreet, minimally invasive devices facilitate continuous monitoring, particularly for patients suffering from chronic diseases.

Advantages and challenges of remote monitoring techniques

New remote monitoring and diagnostic techniques offer numerous **advantages**. They enable **continuous**, reactive **monitoring**, with real-time data facilitating **early detection of complications**. This translates into reduced hospital stays, optimized treatment and an overall improvement in patients' quality of life. For healthcare professionals, these technologies offer greater access to patient health information, reinforcing **medical decision-making**.

However, these innovations also pose **challenges**. One of the main issues is **data management**. The sheer volume of data collected by these devices requires a robust infrastructure to ensure storage, analysis and security. The protection of patients' **personal data**, while respecting confidentiality, is also a major concern, especially with the rise of digital health platforms.

Another challenge lies in the **accessibility of technologies**. Although connected devices are becoming increasingly commonplace, their cost remains an obstacle for some patients, particularly in areas where access to care and technology is limited. It is therefore essential that these innovations are accompanied by measures to **reduce inequalities in access** to care.

Chapter 9

The work environment and risk prevention in gastroenterology

1 Managing infectious risks: a daily challenge

• Preventing nosocomial infections in gastroenterology
Preventing **nosocomial infections** in gastroenterology is of vital importance for the safety of hospitalized patients and the quality of the care they receive. These infections, contracted during a hospital stay, can occur in all care departments, but the field of gastroenterology presents particularities that increase the risk of infection. Patients with gastrointestinal diseases, who are often immunocompromised or require endoscopic procedures, are more vulnerable to infection. In addition, frequent medical manipulation of the digestive tract, the use of probes and catheters, and endoscopic procedures all contribute to the risk of infection. It is therefore essential to implement strict and rigorous preventive measures to minimize these risks and protect patients.

The main nosocomial infections in gastroenterology

In gastroenterology, the most frequent nosocomial infections are those **linked to invasive devices** (central venous catheters, nasogastric tubes, drains), as well as those contracted during **endoscopic procedures**. Infections can be bacterial, viral or fungal in origin, and affect various organs of the digestive system.

Catheter-related infections

Nasogastric tubes and central venous catheters are commonly used to feed, administer treatments or drain the digestive tract. However, their use presents an increased risk of nosocomial infections, particularly if the devices are poorly maintained or if aseptic procedures are not followed. These infections can affect the digestive tract, but can also lead to serious **septicemia** in the event of bacterial contamination.

Post-endoscopic infections

Endoscopic procedures (gastroscopy, colonoscopy, endoscopic retrograde cholangiopancreatography - ERCP) are frequent interventions in gastroenterology to diagnose or treat pathologies. If performed incorrectly, or if instruments are insufficiently disinfected, they can introduce pathogens into the digestive tract. Nosocomial post-endoscopic infections include bacterial **infections** such as **Clostridioides difficile** (C. difficile), and infections by multi-resistant agents.

Infections associated with immunosuppression

Many gastroenterology patients suffer from **chronic inflammatory bowel disease** (IBD), such as Crohn's disease or ulcerative colitis. These patients are often under immunosuppressive treatment (corticosteroids, biotherapies), which puts them at greater risk of nosocomial infections, including **fungal** or viral **infections** (herpes, cytomegalovirus). Preventing these infections requires increased attention, particularly in terms of hygiene and monitoring for signs of infection.

Measures to prevent nosocomial infections

The prevention of nosocomial infections relies on a combination of **strict hygiene** measures, **aseptic** procedures, **ongoing training of** nursing **staff**, and **active** infection **surveillance**. In gastroenterology, prevention must be adapted to the specific features of the department and the types of patients under its care.

Hand hygiene and aseptic gestures

Hand hygiene remains one of the simplest and most effective measures for preventing nosocomial infections. It is essential that all caregivers scrupulously respect hand-washing protocols before and after every patient contact, as well as before any invasive procedure or handling of medical devices. The use of **hydro-alcoholic solutions** is recommended, as they enable rapid and effective disinfection, thus reducing the risk of pathogen transmission.

Aseptic procedures must also be observed when handling invasive devices such as nasogastric tubes, venous catheters and drains. Any insertion or handling of these devices must be carried out under rigorous aseptic conditions, using sterile equipment and appropriate techniques to prevent the introduction of germs.

Disinfection of endoscopic instruments

In gastroenterology, **endoscope** disinfection is a critical factor in preventing nosocomial infections. These instruments are reused from patient to patient, and must undergo a strict disinfection procedure after each use. Disinfection must be carried out in several stages, including mechanical cleaning to remove organic debris, followed by high-level chemical disinfection.

Disinfection procedures must be regularly audited and validated to ensure their effectiveness. **Automation** of endoscope cleaning and disinfection processes is also encouraged to minimize human error and ensure complete instrument sterilization.

Precautions with invasive devices

Invasive devices such as **probes, drains and catheters** represent potential entry points for infection. It is therefore crucial to limit their use to what is strictly necessary, and to remove them as soon as their function is no longer essential. When they are in place, daily monitoring of the insertion site is necessary to detect early signs of infection (redness, warmth, discharge) or local complications.

Caregivers should also ensure that **dressings** around catheters or probes **are changed regularly**, and follow specific protocols for administering nutrients or drugs via these devices to prevent contamination.

Monitoring and isolation of infected patients

Active surveillance of nosocomial infections enables us to detect cases of infection at an early stage and take the necessary measures to limit their spread. This surveillance is based on the implementation of infection **reporting** systems, with regular epidemiological analysis to identify sources of infection and areas at risk within the hospital.

In gastroenterology departments, it is often necessary to take **isolation measures** for patients carrying contagious pathogens, such as C. difficile infections, or multi-resistant agents. Isolation limits the spread of these germs to other patients and nursing staff. Individual rooms and specific protocols (gloves, masks, gowns) must be respected when caring for these patients.

Ongoing training and a culture of prevention

Ongoing training of healthcare staff is essential to ensure effective prevention of nosocomial infections. Teams must be trained in **best hygiene practices**, techniques for handling invasive devices, and protocols for disinfecting medical equipment.

Infection prevention awareness must also be part of the department culture. Encouraging staff to report non-conformities, respect barrier procedures, and keep abreast of new recommendations is essential to instilling a culture of safety and infectious risk prevention.

- Asepsis techniques and hand hygiene: a crucial reminder

Aseptic techniques and **hand hygiene** are essential pillars of infection prevention in the hospital environment, including gastroenterology. These practices are essential to guarantee patient safety and reduce the transmission of nosocomial infections. Although their importance is widely recognized, regular reminders of these techniques are crucial to maintaining high standards of care and effectively combating infections. Every care procedure, however simple, must be carried out in strict compliance with hygiene and asepsis measures to protect patients and caregivers alike.

Hand hygiene: a simple but vital gesture

Hand hygiene is the simplest and most effective measure for preventing the transmission of infections in a medical environment. Hand washing or disinfection eliminates the majority of potentially pathogenic micro-organisms that caregivers may acquire through contact with patients, surfaces or medical instruments. However, compliance with this procedure is sometimes inadequate, leading to more frequent nosocomial infections. A regular reminder of the importance and good practice of hand hygiene is therefore essential.

When should you practice hand hygiene?

The **World Health Organization (WHO)** has defined five crucial times when hand hygiene should be practiced in a medical setting:

1. **Before any contact with the patient**: To prevent transmission of germs to the patient from the caregiver's hands.
2. **Before an aseptic procedure**: When handling sterile medical equipment, administering invasive care (catheter insertion, catheter catheterization), or preparing medication.

3. **After a risk of exposure to biological fluids**: for example, after touching blood, secretions, excretions or soiled dressings.
4. **After touching the patient**: To avoid transferring germs from one patient to another or to the hospital environment.
5. **After touching the patient's environment**: This includes surfaces and objects around the patient, such as medical equipment, bed linen or bedroom furniture.

By respecting these five moments, nursing staff can considerably reduce the spread of nosocomial infections.

Hand-washing techniques

There are two main methods of ensuring good hand hygiene: **washing with soap and water**, and the **use of hydro-alcoholic solutions** (SHA). Each method has its own specific indications, and must be carried out with care to ensure optimum elimination of germs.

1. **Hand washing with soap and water**: This procedure is recommended when hands are visibly dirty, soiled with biological fluids or after caring for patients infected with resistant agents. Hand washing should last at least **40 to 60 seconds** and include thorough cleaning of all areas: palms, backs of hands, interdigital spaces, thumbs, fingertips and wrists. Hands should be dried with a single-use paper towel, and the faucet closed with the towel to prevent recontamination.

2. **Disinfection with hydro-alcoholic solution**: In most situations, the use of SHA is faster and just as effective as conventional washing, provided that hands are not visibly soiled. Rubbing should last **20 to 30 seconds** and follow a standardized procedure to include all parts of the hand. The advantage of SHA is that it is readily available and can be used between treatments without leaving the patient's room.

Asepsis techniques: the barrier against infection

Asepsis techniques are a set of procedures designed to prevent the introduction of micro-organisms into a sterile area or onto medical devices. In gastroenterology, where invasive devices such as probes, catheters and endoscopes are frequently used, compliance with asepsis rules is essential to reduce the risk of infection.

Basic principles of asepsis

Asepsis involves maintaining the **sterility of** instruments and surfaces used in invasive care. The main aim is to avoid contamination by pathogenic organisms-micro, which may be present in the environment, on the hands of caregivers or on the patient's skin.

1. **Washing hands and wearing gloves**: Before any invasive procedure, such as nasogastric tube insertion, catheter placement or endoscopy, hand hygiene must be carried out as recommended. **Sterile gloves** must then be worn, especially for any procedure involving contact with sterile medical devices or areas of the body normally protected from the outside world.

2. **Preparation of the operating field**: The area where the invasive procedure is to be performed must be carefully prepared with an **antiseptic** (e.g. chlorhexidine or iodized alcohol solution), and covered with sterile drapes to avoid external contamination. The patient's skin should be disinfected by cleaning in a circular motion from the center outwards, to reduce the microbial load.

3. **Use of sterile materials**: All materials used in invasive procedures, such as catheters, probes, needles or infusion sets, must be **sterile**. Packages must be opened aseptically,

272

avoiding any contact with the outside of the pack. What's more, if the procedure is long or complex, it's imperative to check regularly that the sterile field is maintained and that the equipment has not been accidentally contaminated.

4. **Disinfection of reusable devices**: In gastroenterology, devices such as **endoscopes** or biopsy instruments are reused after each patient. Their disinfection must follow rigorous protocols to eliminate all traces of micro-organisms. Mechanical cleaning precedes high-level chemical disinfection, and compliance with these steps is essential to prevent cross-transmission of infections.

Ongoing training and daily vigilance

Maintaining hand hygiene and asepsis techniques relies on the **daily vigilance** of care staff, and on **ongoing training** to ensure that everyone is up to date with best practice. Nosocomial infections often occur as a result of negligence or fatigue, so it's essential to incorporate regular reminders and checks on compliance with hygiene procedures into caregivers' routines.

Healthcare facilities can organize **regular training sessions**, internal audits and practical workshops to reinforce the culture of asepsis and the importance of hand hygiene. It is also crucial to **monitor the supply of** hydro-alcoholic solutions, sterile gloves and disinfection equipment to ensure that caregivers always have access to the tools they need to comply with hygiene rules.

• Care of immunocompromised patients: specific precautions

Care of immunocompromised patients requires a particularly rigorous and attentive approach, as these patients are much more vulnerable to infections than the general population. Immunodepression, whether caused by chronic diseases (such as HIV or cancer), treatments (chemotherapy, immunosuppressants, corticosteroids) or genetic conditions, weakens the body's natural defenses, making it difficult to fight pathogens. Specific precautions in their management are essential to minimize the risk of infections, which can be serious, even fatal, in this context. This involves **reinforced hygiene measures**, **continuous monitoring** for signs of infection, and **adaptation of care to** prevent unnecessary exposure to infectious agents.

Reinforced hygiene measures

Immunocompromised patients are extremely susceptible to nosocomial and opportunistic infections, which is why **hygiene** is an essential pillar of their care. Standard hygiene measures must be strictly applied, and sometimes reinforced, to limit any risk of contamination.

Hand hygiene

Hand hygiene is the most crucial measure in preventing infections in immunocompromised patients. Nursing staff, visitors and even patients must wash their hands rigorously and frequently, for every direct or indirect contact. The use of **hydro-alcoholic solutions** is preferred, as they are both effective and easy to apply between treatments. Hand washing with soap and water is essential after any contact with biological fluids, or when hands are visibly dirty.

Wearing personal protective equipment

Wearing **gloves**, **masks** and sometimes **gowns** is often necessary when caring for immunocompromised patients, especially if staff come into contact with biological fluids or if there is a risk of transmitting pathogens. This personal protective equipment must be used according to strict protocols and disposed of after each treatment, to avoid any risk of cross-contamination.

Environmental control

The immunocompromised patient's environment must be kept as **sterile** as possible, or at least at low risk of infection. This includes regular cleaning and disinfection of surfaces and medical equipment. **Single rooms** are often necessary for these patients to limit their exposure to infections from other patients or nursing staff. Rooms must be cleaned according to specific protocols, using appropriate disinfectants.

In addition, additional measures can be taken to control **air quality**, including the use of HEPA air filters in certain care units, particularly for patients undergoing treatments such as bone marrow transplants, which expose them to the risk of fungal infections.

Enhanced clinical monitoring

In immunocompromised patients, infections can develop rapidly and silently, without the classic signs (fever, redness, pain). **Increased surveillance** is therefore essential to detect any deterioration in health status at an early stage.

Monitoring for signs of infection

Caregivers must be particularly attentive **to atypical signs of infection**. For example, fever, often an early sign of infection, may be absent in patients on immunosuppressive therapy. Slight alterations in vital parameters, such as increased respiratory or heart rate, may be early indicators of an underlying infection. Any change in clinical status (fatigue, confusion, unexplained pain, loss of appetite) should be reported and managed immediately.

Opportunistic infections, which affect these patients at a stage when their immune defenses are weakened, are often caused by pathogens that would not affect a healthy person, such as certain bacteria, viruses (herpes, cytomegalovirus), or fungi (aspergillosis, candidiasis). **Regular** biological **monitoring**

)blood counts, blood cultures) is also crucial for early detection of infection before clinical signs appear.

Monitoring invasive devices

Invasive medical devices, such as **central venous catheters**, **urinary catheters** or **nasogastric tubes**, are potential entry points for infections in immunocompromised patients. These devices should be used only when necessary, and their handling should follow **strict aseptic** rules. Insertion sites should be monitored daily for redness, pain, discharge or other signs of local infection.

Special precautions for specific care

Care of immunocompromised patients often involves **adaptations** to minimize the risk of infection, whether in terms of treatment, nutritional management or prevention of complications.

Prevention of opportunistic infections

Immunocompromised patients, especially those undergoing chemotherapy or biological therapies, are at increased risk of **opportunistic infections**. **Antimicrobial prophylaxis** (antibiotics, antifungals, antivirals) is therefore often necessary, depending on the patient's specific infectious risk. For example, transplant patients may receive antibiotics to prevent pneumocystis jirovecii lung infections, or antivirals to prevent herpes reactivation.

Nutritional management

Nutrition plays a crucial role in the management of immunocompromised patients. Patients undergoing chemotherapy or suffering from chronic gastrointestinal diseases may suffer from malnutrition, which further weakens their immune systems. A **safe diet**, often free from raw or undercooked products, is recommended to limit the risk of introducing bacteria or parasites into the body.

If enteral or parenteral nutrition is required, probes or catheters must be handled with strict aseptic precautions, and nutrition bags must be prepared under sterile conditions to avoid contamination.

Patient and family education

Immunocompromised patients and their relatives need to be **informed and trained** on the precautions to be taken to avoid infection. This includes advice on hand hygiene, respiratory hygiene (wearing a mask if necessary), and visiting management. In some cases, restrictions on visiting can be put in place to reduce exposure to pathogens.

Patients should also be aware of the signs of infection to look out for at home, and know when to consult their doctor promptly. Education also covers prophylactic treatment and the importance of scrupulously following the recommendations of their healthcare team.

Protective isolation

In some cases, it may be necessary to institute **protective isolation** for immunocompromised patients, particularly in the most critical phases of their treatment, such as after bone marrow transplantation. Isolation is designed to protect the patient from any potential source of infection. Rooms are specially equipped to maintain a low-germ environment, with **HEPA air filters** and rigorous disinfection protocols.

2 Safety at work: protecting caregivers and patients

- Safe handling of heavy patients: avoiding musculoskeletal disorders

The **safe handling of heavy patients** is a major issue in healthcare establishments, as it involves the health and safety of both patients and caregivers. Lifting, mobilizing or repositioning a heavy patient can involve considerable physical effort for care assistants and nurses, leading to significant risks of **musculoskeletal disorders (MSDs)**. These disorders, which mainly affect the back, shoulders and upper limbs, are a frequent cause of work stoppage in the healthcare sector. It is therefore essential to implement appropriate techniques for handling these patients, while preserving the physical integrity of caregivers and guaranteeing patient safety.

Understanding the risks of MSDs among caregivers

Musculoskeletal disorders are conditions that affect joints, muscles, tendons or nerves as a result of repetitive movements or excessive effort. In the hospital environment, MSDs are mainly caused by inappropriate movements or the frequent handling of heavy loads, in this case patients who need help to get up, turn around or change position.

The main causes of MSDs among caregivers include :

- **Sudden** or inappropriate **movements** when moving patients;
- **Carrying excessive loads**, particularly where there is a lack of personnel or suitable equipment;
- **Uncomfortable** or prolonged **postures**, such as bending or squatting to lift a patient;
- **Repetitive movements** without breaks or alternating tasks, such as repositioning bedridden patients.

The areas most affected are generally the **back**, especially the lumbar spine, as well as the **shoulders** and **knees**, due to forced postures and sustained effort.

Basic principles of safe patient handling

To prevent musculoskeletal disorders, it is crucial to follow **safe handling** principles. These principles aim to limit physical effort and protect the caregiver's joints and muscles, while ensuring the patient's comfort and safety.

Pre-evaluation

Before any manipulation, it is essential to assess the situation, taking into account the patient's weight, height and physical capabilities. This assessment determines whether repositioning or lifting can be carried out manually, or whether the use of **mechanical aids** or **specific techniques** is necessary. It's important never to underestimate the load a patient represents, even if he or she seems cooperative.

It is also essential to **communicate with the patient** before handling, to ensure understanding and cooperation. Patients can sometimes contribute to their own mobility by actively participating in the movement, thus reducing the burden on the caregiver.

Use of ergonomic postures

When handling a patient, adopting **ergonomic postures** is essential to reduce the risk of injury.

1. **Keep your back straight**: It's important to keep your back straight at all times and avoid bending forward. Repeated bending or twisting of the spine can lead to muscle or joint damage.
2. **Bend the knees**: To lift or reposition a patient, caregivers must bend their knees, using mainly leg muscles rather

than back muscles. This maintains a stable posture and distributes the effort over stronger, less vulnerable muscles.

3. **Proximity to the patient**: The caregiver should remain as close as possible to the patient during handling to avoid the leverage effect which increases the load on the back and shoulders.

4. **Coordinating movements**: When several caregivers are involved, it is crucial to coordinate movements to avoid unbalanced efforts. Clear instructions and teamwork help to reduce the physical load for everyone involved.

Use of technical and mechanical aids

To reduce physical strain, it is essential to use appropriate **technical aids**, particularly when handling heavy or non-autonomous patients. Mechanical equipment can be used to lift, move or reposition patients, reducing the manual effort required of caregivers.

1. **Patient lifts: Mechanical or electric patient lifts** are devices designed to lift a patient from bed to a chair, or to reposition the patient in bed. They considerably reduce the physical effort required for lifting, while guaranteeing patient safety. The use of this equipment requires appropriate training to ensure correct and safe operation.

2. **Glide sheets: Glide sheets** or glide systems facilitate lateral transfers or repositioning in bed. They reduce friction and the effort required to turn or straighten a patient, thus limiting strain on caregivers' backs and shoulders.

3. **Positioning cushions: Ergonomic cushions** can be used to reposition patients safely, distributing body weight evenly and avoiding sudden movements. These cushions also help keep the patient in a comfortable posture, reducing the need for frequent handling.

4. **Grab bars and mobilization aids**: Installing **grab bars** or other support devices around the bed or in the bathroom can enable patients to actively participate in their movements. These technical aids promote autonomy and reduce muscular strain for caregivers.

Training and teamwork

One of the keys to preventing musculoskeletal disorders lies in **training** nursing staff in good handling practices. Regular training in lifting techniques, handling of technical aids and ergonomic postures all help to anchor safe behavior.

Moreover, **teamwork** is essential when handling heavy patients. It's often safer and more efficient to mobilize several caregivers for the same movement, rather than leave the lifting or repositioning to a single professional. Cooperation helps to spread the load and limit the risk of injury. **Briefings** before each complex mobilization can help coordinate efforts and ensure that everyone is aligned with the procedure to be followed.

Adapting the environment to facilitate handling

Space planning is a crucial factor in the safe handling of heavy patients. Patient rooms must be designed to allow easy access to care equipment and mechanical aids. A height-adjustable bed, for example, enables the caregiver to adapt his or her posture to the handling task in hand, thus reducing physical strain. Similarly, adapted chairs with mechanisms to facilitate sitting or standing up can reduce the number of manual interventions required.

Monitoring for signs of MSD and pain management

Despite the application of the best handling techniques, caregivers need to be alert to **early signs of musculoskeletal disorders**, such as back pain, shoulder tension or joint stiffness. Early treatment is essential to prevent MSDs from worsening. In the event of pain or discomfort, it is important to report these symptoms immediately and adapt tasks accordingly to avoid repeated overload.

Pain management through stretching exercises, muscle strengthening, or consultations with a physiotherapist can help prevent RSI and keep staff in good health.

- • Use of personal protective equipment (PPE) in gastroenterology

The **use of personal protective equipment (PPE)** in gastroenterology is essential to protect both caregivers and patients from infection and contamination. This department, which focuses on the diagnosis and treatment of disorders of the digestive system, often exposes staff to pathogens transmitted by bodily fluids such as stool, blood and gastrointestinal secretions. In addition, frequent procedures such as endoscopies, biopsies and the handling of invasive devices increase the risk of contact with potentially infectious biological substances. The use of PPE is therefore a key element in the prevention of nosocomial infections and the reduction of occupational risks.

Role of PPE in gastroenterology

Personal protective equipment (PPE) is a device or garment designed to protect healthcare professionals from direct exposure to hazardous or infectious substances. In gastroenterology, where caregivers are frequently in contact with patients likely to carry pathogens, PPE forms an essential barrier against infection. Their use is particularly crucial during invasive procedures such as digestive endoscopies, where there is a high risk of contamination by body fluids.

PPE comprises several elements, such as **gloves**, **gowns**, **masks** (including respirators), **goggles**, and sometimes **face shields** or **overshoes**. Each piece of equipment has a specific role, and their combined use in high-risk environments, such as the endoscopic unit, provides optimum protection.

282

The different types of PPE and their use in gastroenterology

Depending on the specific procedures and risks encountered, the use of PPE may vary. It is important to select the appropriate equipment according to the nature of the care provided, the type of contact with body fluids, and the degree of protection required.

Gloves

Gloves are a basic piece of equipment in gastroenterology. They are used in almost all care situations where the caregiver is likely to come into contact with bodily fluids or potentially contaminated surfaces. In gastroenterology, gloves are indispensable when handling **endoscopes** and probes, or when administering care to patients with gastrointestinal infections.

Gloves must **be single-use**, discarded after each contact with the patient or his environment, and replaced immediately if torn. It is essential to choose gloves suited to the nature of the care: **sterile gloves are** required for invasive procedures, while **non-sterile gloves** may suffice for routine care or handling without risk of direct contamination.

Blouses

Protective gowns are essential to protect nursing staff's clothing and skin from splashes of body fluids. In gastroenterology, they are particularly used during procedures where the risk of splashing is high, such as **endoscopies**, **biopsy sampling** or interventions involving invasive devices. Gowns must be worn appropriately, with full closure at the back, and removed carefully to avoid contamination from outside the gown.

Depending on requirements, **disposable** or **washable gowns** can be used. Where the risk of contamination is high, single-use gowns made of impermeable material are recommended.

283

Masks and respirators

Surgical masks and **respirators** (such as FFP2 or N95) play a key role in protecting the respiratory tract. In gastroenterology, caregivers are exposed to risks of **airborne** or **droplet transmission**, particularly during procedures where gastrointestinal secretions may be aerosolized, such as during gastroscopy or bronchial endoscopy.

Surgical masks protect primarily against droplets, while **FFP2** or N95 **masks** offer enhanced protection against potentially infectious aerosols. They are used during high-risk procedures, particularly in situations where patients may be carriers of respiratory-transmitted infectious diseases (such as **Clostridioides difficile**, or certain gastrointestinal viral infections).

Goggles and face shields

Goggles or **face shields** are needed to protect the eyes and face from splashes of body fluids, which can occur during procedures such as colonoscopy or gastroscopy. This equipment is essential to prevent contamination of ocular mucous membranes by pathogens transmitted by bodily fluids, and is often combined with the wearing of masks to ensure complete coverage of possible routes of entry for infections.

Face shields can also protect against larger splashes, particularly in aerosol-generating procedures or when using devices such as endoscopic suction machines.

Overshoes and hats

Although less frequently used than other PPE, **overshoes** and **caps** may be required in highly controlled environments, such as operating theatres or sterile procedure rooms, to prevent cross-contamination from footwear or hair.

Key times for wearing PPE in gastroenterology

The use of PPE must be **systematic** and adapted to the specific risks of each procedure. In gastroenterology, several key moments require particular attention:

1. **Endoscopic procedures**: When performing gastroscopy, colonoscopy or ERCP, caregivers are exposed to digestive fluids potentially containing infectious agents. Wearing gloves, surgical or FFP2 masks, goggles or face shields, as well as gowns, is essential to protect against splashes and droplets.

2. **Handling invasive devices**: The insertion or removal of **nasogastric tubes**, **drains** or catheters also **requires** specific precautions. Gloves, and sometimes gowns and masks, are required to prevent contamination of the caregiver and limit the risk of infection to the patient.

3. **Care of infected patients**: Patients with gastrointestinal infections, such as **Clostridioides difficile** infections, require enhanced precautions to prevent the spread of pathogens. The wearing of full PPE (gloves, gowns, masks) is crucial, combined with strict isolation measures to minimize the risk of transmission.

PPE removal and disposal

Just as important as wearing PPE, but often overlooked, is **removing** and **disposing of** it. PPE must be carefully removed to avoid contamination through contact with the outside of gloves, gowns or masks. Precise gestures must be followed, starting by removing gloves without touching the skin, removing the gown so as not to touch the contaminated outer surface, then removing the goggles and mask last.

Single-use PPE must be disposed of in specific biohazard waste garbage cans, in accordance with infectious waste management protocols. As for reusable equipment (such as safety goggles), they must be disinfected after each use with suitable solutions to guarantee their safety the next time they are used.

Training and vigilance

Staff training in the **correct use of PPE** is essential to ensure optimum protection. Each caregiver must be able to choose the PPE appropriate to the situation, put it on correctly, and remove it while respecting hygiene rules to avoid cross-contamination. Daily vigilance in the use of PPE helps to establish a **culture of safety** in the gastroenterology department, protecting both caregivers and patients.

- Managing the risks of exposure to body fluids (digestive bleeding, vomiting)

Managing the **risks of exposure to body fluids**, such as digestive bleeding and vomiting, is a priority in gastroenterology. These fluids, often carrying bacteria, viruses or other pathogens, can easily contaminate caregivers and surfaces, increasing the risk of transmission of nosocomial infections. Digestive bleeding, vomiting and other digestive excretions are an integral part of care in this area, and therefore require particular vigilance. Management of these risks relies on a combination of **preventive measures**, **personal protective equipment (PPE)** and **education** of healthcare staff to ensure the safety of patients and caregivers.

Understanding the risks associated with body fluids in gastroenterology

Patients undergoing gastroenterology care are often subject to **digestive disorders** that can lead to **bleeding** or **vomiting**, particularly in the context of serious gastrointestinal diseases such as ulcers, esophageal varices, digestive cancers or chronic inflammatory bowel disease (IBD). These episodes can release body fluids containing infectious agents, such as bacteria (e.g.

Clostridioides difficile), liver viruses (hepatitis B or C), or gastrointestinal parasites.

The risk for caregivers is linked to **contamination by direct contact** with these fluids, but also to exposure to **droplets** or **aerosols** produced during vomiting or the management of active bleeding. If these fluids come into contact with **mucous membranes** or **injured skin**, or are inhaled in the form of aerosols, they can transmit potentially serious infections. It is therefore essential to follow strict protocols to limit such exposure.

Protective measures in the event of digestive tract haemorrhage

Digestive bleeding is a frequent occurrence in gastroenterology, and can manifest itself as vomiting blood (hematemesis), rectal bleeding (rectorrhagia) or the presence of digested blood in the stool (melena). These situations, which can be critical, require rapid and effective management, while protecting caregivers from the risks of exposure.

Wearing personal protective equipment (PPE)

Wearing **PPE** is the first line of defense against exposure to body fluids during digestive bleeding. **Gloves, gowns, masks** and **goggles** or **face shields** are essential to protect the skin, mucous membranes and respiratory tract of caregivers.

1. **Gloves**: They must be worn whenever the patient or body fluids come into contact with them. **Sterile gloves** are recommended for invasive procedures, while **non-sterile** gloves may be sufficient for less risky manipulations (e.g. perfusion adjustment, monitoring vital parameters).

2. **Gowns: Waterproof gowns** are necessary to prevent contamination of clothing in the event of splashes of blood or other digestive fluids. They must cover the arms and

287

torso completely, and be removed carefully to avoid touching the contaminated exterior.

3. **Masks and goggles**: **Surgical masks** and **goggles** (or face shields) protect against **droplets** and **aerosols** that may be projected when managing a digestive bleed. This equipment is particularly essential when handling the respiratory tract or upper digestive tract, as in emergency endoscopic procedures.

Management of digestive bleeding

When a patient presents with a **digestive bleed**, it's essential to stabilize the condition quickly, while minimizing the risk of exposure for caregivers. A team approach, with well-distributed tasks, enables the situation to be managed in an orderly fashion.

1. **Managing invasive devices**: In the event of active digestive bleeding, devices such as **nasogastric tubes** may be used to evacuate blood or gastrointestinal secretions. **Aseptic precautions** are essential when handling these devices, to avoid cross-contamination and protect the caregiver from splashes.

2. **Precautions during endoscopic procedures**: During **emergency endoscopies**, where it may be necessary to visualize and treat hemorrhage, the risk of splashing blood and fluids is high. In addition to PPE, suitable **suction techniques** must be employed to limit the spread of fluids. Endoscopes and reusable equipment must be disinfected according to strict protocols to prevent transmission of pathogens.

3. **Environmental control**: It is important to **protect the immediate environment** around the patient to limit the spread of fluids. Surfaces must be cleaned and disinfected promptly after any bleeding episode to prevent blood from contaminating other patients or staff.

Vomiting management and aerosol precautions

Vomiting is common in gastroenterology, particularly in patients suffering from intestinal obstruction, severe gastritis or after certain surgical procedures. Vomit may contain infectious agents, and the sprays or aerosols it generates represent a major risk for caregivers.

PPE and respiratory protection

In addition to **impermeable gloves** and **gowns**, **FFP2** or **N95 masks** are particularly recommended when managing patients likely to vomit, especially if they are infected with airborne or fecal-oral pathogens. **Goggles** or **face shields** should be used to prevent splashing in the eyes, a potential route of transmission.

Handling vomiting devices

Devices such as **emesis bags or basins** must be handled with care. Gloves should be changed immediately after handling these devices, and they should be disposed of or cleaned according to biological waste management protocols.

1. **Room ventilation**: When a patient is vomiting, it's crucial to ensure that the room is well **ventilated**, to limit the concentration of aerosols. If possible, air filtration systems should be used, especially in units where several patients share the same room.

2. **Isolating infectious patients**: If a patient is vomiting due to a gastrointestinal infection (e.g. **Clostridioides difficile**), it is essential to **isolate** him or her from other patients to limit the risk of spread. Visitors must also comply with strict hygiene and protection protocols.

Cleaning and waste management

The **management of waste** arising from the care of patients with digestive haemorrhage or vomiting is crucial to prevent the spread of pathogens.

1. **Contaminated waste**: Contaminated **gowns, gloves, masks** and other materials should be disposed of **in infectious waste garbage cans**, not conventional garbage cans. Reusable devices, such as safety goggles, must be thoroughly disinfected with appropriate products after each use.

2. **Surface cleaning**: Surfaces contaminated with blood or vomit should be cleaned immediately with **broad-spectrum disinfectants**, effective against pathogens transmitted by body fluids, including hepatotropic viruses and resistant intestinal bacteria. Disinfectants containing sodium hypochlorite (bleach) are often recommended for high-risk contamination areas.

3 Medical waste management in the gastroenterology department

• Handling and disposal of sharps waste

Handling and disposing of infectious and sharp waste in the hospital environment are critical tasks to ensure the safety of caregivers, patients and cleaning staff. In gastroenterology, where procedures and treatments frequently involve exposure to body fluids, biological tissues and sharp instruments, rigorous waste management is essential. This waste, whether infectious (potentially contaminating contents, such as blood or digestive secretions) or sharp (needles, scalpels, etc.), must be disposed of according to strict protocols to minimize the risk of injuries and nosocomial infections. Compliance with these protocols is essential not only to protect medical staff, but also to prevent the spread of dangerous pathogens in the hospital environment.

Identification of infectious and sharp waste

Infectious waste and **sharps** are classified as **waste from healthcare activities involving infectious risks (DASRI)**. In gastroenterology, this includes :

1. **Infectious waste**: Any material soiled by body fluids (dressings, compresses, gloves, probes, etc.), as well as biological residues (tissue samples, stools, blood). Reusable instruments (such as endoscopes) require strict disinfection after use.
2. **Sharp waste**: **Needles**, **scalpels**, **blades**, and any other single-use medical device involving the risk of cutting or puncturing, such as catheters, fall into this category.

One of the first steps in waste management is the ability to **correctly identify** these two types of waste in order to handle and dispose of them according to the appropriate protocols.

Handling infectious waste

Infectious waste, which may contain transmissible pathogens (such as viruses, bacteria or fungi), requires **careful handling** to avoid cross-contamination or accidental exposure.

Personal protective equipment (PPE)

When handling infectious waste, it's crucial to wear **gloves**, **gowns** and, if necessary, **masks** and **goggles**. This PPE creates a barrier between the caregiver and the contaminated waste, minimizing the risk of exposure through direct contact with body fluids or soiled surfaces. Gloves must be changed after each handling of infectious waste, to prevent any spread.

Suitable bags and containers

Infectious waste must be collected in **specific bags**, often yellow or red in color, designated for DASRI. These bags are designed to resist punctures and leaks. They must be closed properly after use to prevent accidental spillage. It is important never to overfill the bags, as this increases the risk of breakage and contamination.

In units such as gastroenterology, where caregivers may handle waste containing biological fluids, such as nasogastric tubes or blood-soaked dressings, this waste must be placed immediately after use in DASRI bags, without prolonged contact with care surfaces.

Handling sharp waste

Sharps pose a particular risk of injury and direct exposure to pathogens through **accidental bites** or **cuts**. To handle them safely, there are specific practices to be strictly followed.

Use of sharps containers

Needles, scalpel blades, catheters and other sharp instruments must be disposed of immediately after use in **rigid containers** specially designed for sharps waste. These containers, often yellow in color, are leakproof, puncture-resistant and fitted with a secure locking system to prevent accidents. Containers should always be placed close to the treatment site to limit the transport of sharps and minimize the risk of injury during disposal.

It is essential **never to recap needles** after use, as this increases the risk of accidental puncture. Needles must be returned to the container immediately after injection or blood collection.

Precautions when transporting sharp waste

Sharps containers must not be filled beyond their maximum capacity. When three-quarters full, they should be sealed and sent for incineration or special treatment. Containers should be transported carefully, without being overturned, to avoid any risk of leakage or puncture.

Safe disposal of sharps waste

Once waste has been correctly collected and handled, its **disposal** follows strictly regulated procedures to ensure that it no longer poses a threat to public health or the environment.

Infectious waste treatment

Infectious waste generally undergoes specific treatment before disposal. These include **disinfection** or **sterilization processes** (such as autoclaving, which uses pressurized steam to kill pathogens), or **incineration** methods. High-temperature incineration completely destroys the infectious agents present in waste, while reducing the total volume of waste disposed of.

Healthcare establishments are required to work with companies specializing in the treatment of **DASRI**, who collect the filled bags and containers and transport them to approved treatment units. The waste is then treated in accordance with public health and environmental standards.

Sharps waste management

Sharps, once collected in their rigid containers, also undergo a specialized incineration or treatment process to eliminate infectious risks. These containers must be carefully sealed and transported according to specific procedures to avoid exposure during transfer to the treatment units.

Employee training and awareness

Handling and disposing of sharps waste requires **ongoing training** for care teams. Caregivers need to be regularly informed about the risks associated with biological waste and the best practices for handling it safely. This includes reminders of the correct use of PPE, identification of different types of waste, and safe disposal procedures.

Awareness-raising sessions can also be organized for non-healthcare staff, such as cleaners or maintenance workers, who may come into contact with hazardous waste. A good understanding of waste management protocols is essential to prevent accidents and reduce the transmission of infections.

- Compliance with hospital waste sorting protocols

Compliance with hospital waste sorting protocols is essential to ensure the safety of patients, carers and cleaning staff, while protecting the environment. Hospital waste is varied and includes potentially hazardous elements such as biological waste, expired medication, sharp objects and materials contaminated by pathogens. Rigorous waste sorting minimizes the risk of infection, injury and exposure to harmful substances, while facilitating appropriate treatment. Failure to observe these protocols can have serious consequences, ranging from the spread of nosocomial infections to environmental pollution.

Types and classification of hospital waste

The first crucial aspect in complying with hospital waste sorting protocols is a **clear understanding of the different categories** of waste produced in healthcare establishments. Each category requires specific treatment, and correct sorting at source enables the risks associated with its handling and disposal to be effectively managed.

1. **Waste from care activities involving infectious risks (DASRI)**: This is waste that presents an infectious risk, such as waste soiled with blood, body fluids or excretions, as well as biological waste (tissues, samples). Such waste **is** classified as **hazardous** because it can transmit infections or pathogens. It also includes **sharp waste** (needles, scalpels, catheters), which requires specific disposal to avoid injury and contamination.

2. **Non-hazardous medical waste**: This waste does not present an infectious or chemical risk, and includes uncontaminated materials such as packaging, unsoiled gloves, food scraps and paper. This waste is often treated in the same way as household waste, but sorting it is important to avoid any confusion with hazardous waste.

3. **Chemical or toxic waste**: This category includes **expired medicines**, chemicals used in laboratories, disinfectants and other hazardous substances that may be toxic or corrosive. Their handling and disposal require particular vigilance, as they can be harmful to staff and the environment if not properly treated.

4. **Radioactive waste**: This waste, generated during nuclear medicine examinations or radiotherapy treatments, requires very specific treatment because of its long-term hazardousness. Handling and storage must follow rigorous protocols to protect both individuals and the environment.

Importance of sorting at source

Sorting hospital waste at source is a key step in ensuring its safe management. Healthcare staff must be able to **immediately recognize** the nature of the waste produced and place it in the appropriate container, thus avoiding any risk of cross-contamination or dangerous downstream handling. This requires not only **adequate training** for carers and cleaning staff, but also the implementation of collection systems that are easy to use and understand.

Specific containers and clear signage

To facilitate sorting, healthcare establishments must provide **clearly identifiable containers** for each category of waste. **DASRI containers** are generally yellow in color, with specific signage to indicate that they are intended for infectious risk waste. **Sharps containers**, designed to prevent punctures, are often made of rigid plastic, with a small opening to prevent accidental contact. These containers should be distributed throughout all points of care to enable immediate sorting.

Household and non-hazardous **waste** must be disposed of in different-colored bags or containers (often gray or black), separate from medical waste to avoid any confusion. **Chemical waste** must be placed in specific containers, sealed and labeled with the type of product, its hazardousness, and instructions for safe disposal.

Ongoing training and awareness-raising

Compliance with hospital waste sorting protocols also relies on **ongoing** staff **training** and **awareness-raising**. Every employee must be regularly trained in good waste sorting and disposal practices, with reminders of the dangers associated with the mismanagement of certain types of waste. Clear signage near care areas and containers can serve as a reminder of good practice and make it easier to identify different types of waste.

Sorting errors can have serious consequences: infectious waste thrown away with non-hazardous waste can contaminate other materials and endanger clean-up workers, while improperly disposed of sharp waste can cause serious injury.

Safe waste disposal

Once sorted, hospital waste must be **disposed of** appropriately, following specific procedures for each type of waste. Compliance with these protocols is essential to prevent hazardous waste from endangering people or the environment during treatment or transportation.

DASRI: treatment by incineration or disinfection

Hazardous waste (including infectious and sharps waste) generally has to be **incinerated** in specialized units, where high temperatures destroy pathogens and reduce the risk of contamination. Some institutions also use **disinfection processes** prior to incineration, such as autoclaves, which sterilize waste using steam under pressure.

The collection of this waste must be carried out under strict safety conditions, and the bags or containers must be sealed before being transported to approved treatment centers. Needles and sharps containers should never be more than three-quarters full, to avoid accidents, and should be transported with care.

Chemical waste: specialized disposal

Chemical and toxic waste, such as expired medicines and disinfectants, require special disposal. Such waste is often treated by specialized companies who use suitable processes to break down hazardous substances without endangering the environment or human health. For example, chemicals can be neutralized or destroyed in specially adapted facilities before being disposed of.

Household waste: separate management

Once sorted, **non-hazardous waste** follows management routes similar to those for ordinary household waste. It is collected by hospital cleaning services and disposed of in conventional treatment centers, with recycling or landfill processes depending on its nature. It is important not to mix this waste with hazardous waste, to ensure the safety of cleaning staff.

Monitoring and auditing waste management

Compliance with hospital waste sorting protocols should not be limited to initial staff training. **Regular audits** are essential to assess the effectiveness of waste sorting and identify any gaps in the process. These audits enable compliance rates to be measured and inappropriate practices to be quickly corrected. Corrective action may include additional training or changes to the organization of sorting areas.

Healthcare establishments must also keep waste **tracking registers**, to guarantee traceability from source to disposal. This ensures that waste has been treated in accordance with current regulations, and that prompt action can be taken in the event of an incident.

Consequences of non-compliance with protocols

Failure to comply with hospital waste sorting protocols can have **serious consequences**. Inappropriate sorting can put staff at risk of infection or injury, and lead to cross-contamination between hazardous and non-hazardous waste. In addition, it can complicate downstream waste treatment, increasing the risk of environmental pollution and exposure to toxic substances for neighboring communities.

What's more, incorrect sorting can lead to penalties for the healthcare establishment in the event of an inspection by the health authorities. Incidents of non-compliance can damage the institution's reputation, as well as endangering public health.

Chapter 10

The psychological and ethical dimension of gastroenterology care

1 Supporting patients with chronic illnesses

- Managing patients with chronic diseases (Crohn's disease, chronic hepatitis)

Managing patients suffering from chronic diseases such as **Crohn's disease** or **chronic hepatitis** is a major challenge in gastroenterology. These conditions require a multidimensional therapeutic approach, involving continuous care, in-depth patient education and personalized follow-up. Patients with chronic diseases have to cope with long-term treatments, episodes of acute flare-ups and constant lifestyle adjustments. The aim of management is to control symptoms, prevent complications and improve the patient's quality of life.

Characteristics of chronic diseases in gastroenterology

Chronic diseases such as **Crohn's disease** and **chronic hepatitis** profoundly affect patients' lives. Although different in nature, these conditions share a progressive character and a capacity to provoke episodes of relapse interspersed with periods of remission.

1. **Crohn's disease**: This is a chronic inflammatory bowel disease (IBD) that can affect any part of the digestive tract, but generally affects the small intestine and colon. It causes **inflammation** leading to abdominal pain, diarrhea, intense fatigue, and sometimes serious complications such as fistulas or strictures. The disease evolves in **relapses** and remissions, requiring frequent adjustments to treatments.

2. **Chronic hepatitis**: This is characterized by persistent inflammation of the liver, generally caused by viral infections such as **hepatitis B** or **C**, but also by other causes such as alcohol consumption or certain autoimmune diseases. If not properly treated, chronic hepatitis can progress to **cirrhosis** or **liver cancer**.

300

Patients with chronic hepatitis need regular follow-up to prevent these long-term complications.

Care objectives

The management of patients with chronic diseases has several objectives:

- **Relieve symptoms** and improve quality of life;
- **Preventing** long-term **complications**;
- **Prolonging periods of remission**;
- **Educating patients** to take charge of their own health;
- **Adapt treatments** according to disease progression and patient needs.

These objectives require a multidisciplinary approach, involving gastroenterologists, nurses, nutritionists, psychologists and other specialists, depending on the patient's individual needs.

Medical treatment and therapeutic adjustment

The treatment of chronic diseases in gastroenterology often relies on the use of drugs to **control inflammation**, **prevent relapses** and **minimize complications**. In both cases, treatment must be tailored to the severity of symptoms and the patient's response.

Crohn's disease

Treatment of Crohn's disease aims to reduce inflammation and maintain remission for as long as possible. The main classes of drugs used are :

- **Anti-inflammatories** (aminosalicylates) and **corticoids**, to treat inflammatory flare-ups.

- **Immunosuppressants** and **biotherapies**, such as TNF inhibitors (infliximab, adalimumab), which are used to prevent relapses by modulating the immune system.
- **Antibiotics**, to treat infections or complications such as abscesses.

Patient follow-up involves regular monitoring of symptoms, as well as the side-effects of medications, particularly immunosuppressants, which can increase the risk of infection. In the event of stenosis or fistulas, surgery may be required.

Chronic hepatitis

Treatment of chronic hepatitis depends on the underlying cause of the disease.

- Antivirals are the standard treatment for **viral hepatitis** (B or C). Direct antivirals for hepatitis C have revolutionized management, offering high cure rates. For hepatitis B, antivirals such as nucleoside analogues can help control infection, although they do not always cure the disease.
- In cases of **alcoholic** or **autoimmune hepatitis**, cessation of alcohol or the use of corticosteroids and immunosuppressants can stabilize the disease and prevent progression to cirrhosis.

Treatment of chronic hepatitis also includes monitoring for **liver complications** such as cirrhosis, with regular screening for **liver cancer** (ultrasound and alpha-fetoprotein assays) and management of complications such as ascites or liver failure.

Regular monitoring and follow-up

Regular medical follow-up is essential to adapt treatments and monitor the progress of chronic diseases. It includes frequent medical consultations, biological analyses, and sometimes imaging examinations.

1. **Monitoring symptoms and adjusting treatment**: Depending on the response to treatment, the doctor may

adjust the dose of medication, change treatment in the event of resistance or side effects, or decide on additional interventions, such as surgery in the case of Crohn's disease.

2. **Biological monitoring**: blood tests are used to monitor liver parameters (liver enzymes, viral load for viral hepatitis), inflammatory markers (such as CRP in Crohn's disease), and to detect signs of complications, such as anemia or liver failure. These regular check-ups are essential for adjusting treatments and preventing complications.

3. **Imaging and endoscopy**: In Crohn's disease, endoscopies and imaging examinations (MRI, ultrasound) are used to monitor the condition of the intestinal mucosa and detect the formation of strictures, fistulas or cancerous lesions. In the case of chronic hepatitis, regular ultrasound scans are used to monitor the appearance of suspicious nodules that may indicate liver cancer.

Therapeutic education and the active role of the patient

Therapeutic education is a fundamental aspect of the management of patients with chronic diseases. It is essential that patients understand their disease, the objectives of their treatment, and the importance of long-term follow-up. This enables them to manage their symptoms more effectively, adhere to their treatment and play an active role in its management.

1. **Treatment information**: Patients need to understand the benefits of treatments, but also their potential side effects. This includes a clear explanation of the risks and benefits of immunosuppressants or antivirals, and the measures to be taken to avoid complications.

2. **Adapting your lifestyle**: Chronic diseases often involve lifestyle changes. Crohn's disease patients can benefit from tailored dietary advice to avoid irritating foods and prevent flare-ups. For patients suffering from chronic hepatitis, **avoidance of alcohol** and a balanced diet are essential to protect the liver. Smoking cessation and weight management are also recommended to avoid long-term complications.

3. **Recognizing warning signs**: It's important for the patient to be able to recognize the signs of a complication or flare-up (intense abdominal pain, fever, jaundice, extreme fatigue) and to seek prompt medical attention in case of doubt.

Psychological and social support

Chronic diseases have a profound impact on patients' daily lives, both physically and psychologically. Psychological support is essential to help patients cope with the emotional and social challenges of managing a chronic illness.

1. **Managing stress and anxiety**: Crohn's disease flare-ups, for example, can be unpredictable, and uncertainty about the course of the disease can generate stress and anxiety. Psychological support can help patients develop strategies to better manage these emotions.

2. **Social support**: Patient associations, support groups or online exchange platforms can provide **invaluable help** in sharing experiences, getting advice, and breaking the isolation often felt by patients with chronic illnesses.

• Supporting patients in coming to terms with their illness and long-term treatments
Supporting patients in accepting their illness and long-term treatments is a fundamental aspect of gastroenterology care,

particularly for those suffering from chronic diseases such as Crohn's disease, chronic hepatitis, or other digestive disorders. Accepting illness and managing long-term treatment are not immediate processes; they require time, patience and ongoing support from caregivers. Accepting a chronic illness means understanding the limitations it imposes, facing up to uncertainties about how the disease will evolve, and adapting to treatments that are often heavy and restrictive. The role of caregivers is to accompany patients on this journey, to help them live better with their condition.

The challenges of accepting chronic illness

When a patient is diagnosed with a chronic illness, the news is often difficult to accept. Unlike an acute illness, which is resolved in a relatively short space of time, a chronic disease requires lifelong management, with periods of remission and sometimes unpredictable flare-ups. This can generate **feelings of frustration, anger, injustice** and even **depression** in patients.

Patients also have to cope with **changes in their lifestyle**, whether in terms of diet, physical activity or social interactions. Some patients may find it difficult to integrate the restrictions imposed by the disease (such as strict diets or professional adjustments), while others may have difficulty complying with medical treatments, which are often heavy and restrictive.

Acceptance of a chronic illness goes through several phases:

- **Denial**: In the early stages, many patients refuse to accept the disease or minimize its impact, hoping it will go away quickly.
- **Anger and frustration**: the realization that the disease is long-lasting and will affect their daily lives can provoke intense emotional reactions.
- **Negotiation**: Some patients try to find alternatives or solutions to avoid the constraints of their treatment.

- **Depression**: The prospect of having to live with long-term treatments, sometimes with no possible cure, can lead to feelings of discouragement.
- **Acceptance**: With time, and the right support, patients eventually integrate the disease into their lives, adapting their lifestyle and finding ways to manage it as best they can.

The role of caregivers in emotional support

One of the essential roles of caregivers is to **support patients in this process of acceptance**, helping them to understand their disease, encouraging them to express their fears and frustrations, and offering them tools to cope with this new reality. The listening, empathy and presence of caregivers play a crucial role in helping patients overcome the initial shock of diagnosis and gradually adapt to long-term treatments.

Therapeutic education

Therapeutic education is a central pillar in helping patients to accept their illness and become actively involved in their treatment. This education must be personalized, taking into account the patient's level of understanding, concerns and ability to adapt to the new demands of the disease.

1. **Clearly explain the disease and its progression**: A well-informed patient is more likely to accept his or her illness. Caregivers need to explain the nature of the disease, its potential course and the importance of treatment in a way that is easy to understand. For example, in the case of Crohn's disease, explaining inflammatory flare-ups, triggers and treatment objectives can help patients prepare for the ups and downs of the disease.

2. **Deciphering treatments**: Patients need to understand why they are undergoing certain treatments, what the steps are,

and what the expected benefits are. For long-term treatments, such as immunosuppressants or antivirals for chronic hepatitis, it's crucial to stress the importance of **adherence**. Side effects must be discussed in a transparent manner, as must the means of managing them.

Listening and psychological support

Psychological support is essential to help patients overcome the emotionally difficult phases associated with accepting their illness. Support can be provided by a **psychologist** or **psychiatrist**, or by healthcare professionals trained in emotional management. These professionals can help patients identify their fears, verbalize their frustrations, and develop strategies for coping with anxiety or depression.

Patients can also benefit from the **presence of support groups** and associations. Sharing experiences with others in similar situations can help break the isolation often felt in the face of illness, and provide practical advice on how to manage daily life more effectively.

Encouraging autonomy

Once the acceptance phase has begun, it is important to **encourage patients to take charge of their own health**. This involves learning techniques for managing the disease (such as recognizing the signs of flare-ups, adapting one's diet), as well as a degree of autonomy in managing treatment.

Patients need to be involved in decisions concerning their treatment, with the help of their doctor, so that they feel empowered. Enabling them to participate actively in the management of their disease, for example by noting their symptoms or monitoring the evolution of certain biological markers, helps them to better understand their condition and anticipate complications.

Helping patients integrate illness into their daily lives

Chronically ill patients must learn to live with their illness, without making it the center of their lives. This means helping patients to **adapt their daily lives** without feeling that their lives are totally controlled by the disease.

Adapting lifestyle habits

Some chronic diseases, such as Crohn's disease or chronic hepatitis, require adjustments in diet, lifestyle or stress management. Caregivers, with the help of **dieticians** and **nutritionists**, can help patients gradually modify their habits, respecting their preferences and avoiding overly abrupt or restrictive changes.

For Crohn's disease, dietary adjustments may be necessary during flare-ups (residue-free diet, for example), but in periods of remission, a varied and balanced diet should be encouraged to maintain a good quality of life. For chronic hepatitis, it is essential to avoid alcohol and follow appropriate dietary advice to protect the liver.

Maintaining a social and professional life

Acceptance of the disease should not prevent patients from maintaining an **active social life**, and keeping up their professional activity wherever possible. Caregivers can advise adjustments at work (such as flexible hours or job accommodation) to enable patients to remain productive while managing their illness. Encouraging patients to stay involved in social activities and maintain links with those around them is essential to their psychological well-being.

Overcoming discouragement

Patients with chronic illnesses often experience periods of **discouragement**, particularly when the disease worsens or a relapse occurs. It's important for caregivers to adopt a caring and encouraging attitude at these difficult times, reminding them that periods of remission are possible and that treatments can be adjusted to improve quality of life.

Adapting treatments

It is crucial to **regularly reassess** treatments and adjust them if necessary to better meet the patient's needs. This may involve changing treatment, adapting doses, or introducing complementary therapies to relieve certain symptoms (such as pain or fatigue).

Caregivers also need to be attentive to patients' difficulties in adhering to treatment. If side effects are poorly tolerated, or if treatment interferes too much with the patient's quality of life, alternative options can be discussed.

2 Ethical care in gastroenterology: between benevolence and respect for autonomy

- Respecting patient choice in palliative care and invasive treatments

Respect for patient choice in palliative care and invasive treatment is a fundamental principle in medicine, particularly when it comes to the management of chronic or terminal illnesses. In palliative care, the patient is often faced with difficult decisions concerning interventions that could prolong life or relieve symptoms, but which sometimes involve heavy or invasive treatments. These situations require a profound consideration of the patient's values, wishes and quality of life. Respect for the patient's autonomy and preferences is an ethical pillar of modern medicine, and it is essential that caregivers accompany patients in their choices with kindness, without pressure, while guaranteeing clear and complete information.

The caregiver-patient relationship: a respectful dialogue

In palliative care, the role of caregivers is not only to relieve pain and improve quality of life, but also to **actively listen to** the patient's wishes regarding their care. Caregiver-patient dialogue is at the heart of this process, as it enables the patient's priorities to be understood and integrated into medical decisions.

Respect for patient choice is based on open and transparent communication. It is crucial that patients are clearly informed about their state of health, the treatment options available, the expected benefits, and the potential risks. This includes explaining the consequences of each decision, whether to continue an invasive treatment, to refuse an intervention, or to favor palliative care without therapeutic escalation.

Informing without imposing

An essential aspect of respecting patients' choices is to ensure that they have all the **information** they **need** to make an informed decision, while avoiding imposing a medical choice. Caregivers must be careful not to steer a patient's decision towards a course of treatment because of family pressures or medical considerations, without taking the patient's wishes into account. In palliative care, some patients may wish for invasive treatments, such as chemotherapy or palliative surgery, while others prefer a comfort-only approach, even if this means a shorter life expectancy.

Caregivers must therefore :

- **Present options in a neutral way**: Explain the advantages and disadvantages of each approach without imposing a specific medical point of view.
- **Respect the patient's rhythm**: Allow patients the time they need to reflect on their choices, without rushing. Some patients may need several meetings to formulate their wishes or adapt their decision.

Patient autonomy at the heart of decision-making

Autonomy is one of the fundamental ethical principles of medicine. It implies that patients have the right to make decisions about their own health, taking into account their personal values, beliefs and perception of quality of life. This principle is all the more important in palliative care situations, where survival at all costs is not always the primary objective, but where the patient's comfort and dignity become central.

Refusal of treatment

Refusal of treatment is a fundamental right of the patient, even if it may be difficult for caregivers or family to accept. Some patients, whether terminally ill or suffering from advanced chronic illness, may choose not to undergo invasive or aggressive treatment, preferring to let the disease take its natural course. This choice must be **respected**, as long as it is informed and conscientious.

In these situations, it is essential that caregivers :

- **Respect the patient's decision**: While refusing treatment may seem contrary to the medical goal of prolonging life, the patient's choice to prioritize quality of life and refuse invasive procedures must be honored.
- **Accompany the patient in this choice**: Once the patient has made his or her decision, the role of caregivers is to implement measures to ensure the patient's comfort, by

moving towards palliative care adapted to his or her wishes.

Acceptance of invasive treatments

Conversely, some patients may wish to try **invasive treatments** in the hope of prolonging their lives or improving their symptoms, even if the chances of success are low or the risks high. Here too, respect for patient choice is essential. Patients must understand the limits of treatment, its risks, and the potential effects on their quality of life. Once informed, the patient's choice of whether or not to accept these treatments must be taken into account with the same rigor and consideration.

The role of loved ones and caregivers in supporting choices

In palliative care, loved ones often play an important role in decision-making, especially if the patient becomes too debilitated to express him/herself. However, it is essential that the patient's wishes remain at the heart of all decisions, and that their loved ones are **guided** and **supported** in understanding and respecting their choices.

Supporting the family

Relatives may sometimes be tempted to insist on more aggressive treatments or, on the contrary, to stop certain interventions, basing their decisions on their own emotions or beliefs. Caregivers must :

- **Facilitate calm dialogue** between patients and their families, so that everyone understands the patient's real wishes.
- **Ensuring the primacy of the patient's wishes**, even if this may be difficult for relatives to accept.
- **Provide emotional support** to families, who may feel helpless or powerless in the face of their patient's

suffering. Reassure them that respecting the patient's choices is the best way to honor them and guarantee their dignity.

Anticipating and respecting advance directives

The use of **advance directives** is an important step that enables patients to clearly express their wishes concerning their end-of-life or the treatments they accept or refuse. These documents, drawn up in advance when the patient is still in full possession of his or her faculties, help avoid ethical dilemmas in the event of a deterioration in health.

Caregivers must :

- **Encourage patients** to draw up advance directives as soon as possible.
- **Scrupulously respect these directives** if the patient becomes incapable of expressing his or her wishes. This ensures that the patient's choices are respected, even in the absence of an active decision.

Promoting a dignified and peaceful end to life

In palliative care, respect for patient choice is not limited to the question of invasive treatments. It also encompasses **end-of-life** preferences, such as the place of death (at home or in an institution), the type of care received, or the way symptoms are managed (for example, pain management with opioid treatments).

Pain and symptom management

Pain management is a central aspect of palliative care, and each patient may have preferences regarding the level of sedation desired. Some may choose light sedation to remain conscious and lucid for as long as possible, while others may prefer more aggressive pain management, even if it means being deeply sedated. Here again, it is crucial that caregivers :

- **Discuss symptom management options** with the patient.
- **Respect the patient's wishes** in terms of comfort and lucidity.

Respect for dignity

Respecting patients' choices at the end of life also means guaranteeing their **dignity**. This means providing care that is adapted to the patient's comfort (hygiene, nutrition, psychological support), and ensuring that the patient is treated with respect until the end. Caregivers must also respect the patient's spiritual or cultural values, integrating their religious or philosophical preferences into their care.

- The dilemma of artificial nutrition: ethical aspects and the role of the caregiver

The **dilemma of artificial nutrition** is a frequent issue in palliative care and gastroenterology, particularly when patients are in situations where they can no longer feed themselves. This type of nutrition, whether **enteral** (via gastric tube) or **parenteral** (via intravenous infusion), enables essential nutrients to be maintained for patients unable to feed themselves orally. However, the decision to initiate or continue artificial nutrition raises complex **ethical issues**, particularly when the patient's quality of life deteriorates or when he or she is terminally ill. In this context, **the role of the caregiver** is central, both in providing the technical care associated with artificial nutrition and in accompanying patients and their families through this delicate ordeal.

Ethical issues surrounding artificial nutrition

Artificial nutrition, although a technical solution for ensuring the nutrition of patients unable to feed themselves, raises profound **ethical dilemmas**, especially at the end of life or in severe chronic illnesses. These ethical issues revolve around the **appropriateness of treatment, respect for the patient's wishes,** and **quality of life**. The main ethical issues are as follows:

314

Prolonging life or prolonging suffering?

One of the main dilemmas is whether artificial nutrition contributes to **prolonging life** or **prolonging suffering**. In some cases, such as in terminally ill patients, artificial nutrition may prolong survival, but not improve quality of life. For seriously ill or terminally ill patients, artificial nutrition can sometimes be perceived as a **therapeutic escalation** that merely prolongs a situation of suffering, rather than enabling a peaceful end to life. On the other hand, in certain cases of rehabilitation or recovery from acute illness, artificial nutrition can be temporarily beneficial, enabling better recovery.

Respecting patient autonomy

Respect for patient **autonomy** is a fundamental principle of medical ethics. The patient has the right to decide whether or not to receive artificial nutrition. If the patient is still capable of expressing himself, his wishes must be taken into account, whether to accept or refuse artificial nutrition. If the patient is no longer able to express him/herself, **advance directives** or the family's decision must guide the treatment.

Respecting autonomy can be particularly difficult when the patient's wishes are not clearly expressed. In such cases, the decision to start or stop artificial nutrition is based on a **benefit-risk balance**, taking into account the patient's presumed wishes and values. The question of whether artificial nutrition is essential **basic care** or optional **medical treatment** is an ongoing debate in the medical community, with answers varying according to clinical situations and ethical convictions.

Quality of life versus quantity of life

When making decisions about artificial nutrition, the notion of **quality of life** is paramount. Artificially maintaining a nutrient supply can prolong life, but it can also lead to a **reduced quality of life**, notably by creating dependencies on machines, risks of infection, or discomfort linked to the presence of medical devices such as catheters or infusions. In palliative care, the aim is often to prioritize comfort and dignity over prolonging life at all costs. It is therefore crucial to assess whether artificial nutrition actually improves the patient's condition, or merely prolongs an already deteriorating situation.

The caregiver's role in setting up and managing artificial nutrition

The caregiver plays an **essential role** in the day-to-day management of artificial nutrition, both technically and in terms of relationships. They are often the **first** point of **contact** with the patient and family, monitoring the devices and providing invaluable support for the patient's comfort and well-being.

Technical management of artificial nutrition

On a technical level, the caregiver is responsible for several aspects of the management of artificial nutrition, whether enteral or parenteral.

1. **Monitoring probes and devices**: In the case of **enteral nutrition**, the caregiver is responsible for ensuring that the nasogastric tube or gastrostomy is correctly positioned, that it does not move, and that there are no complications such as irritation or infection at the insertion point. He must also report any discomfort or pain expressed by the patient in connection with the tube. For **parenteral nutrition**, he/she monitors infusions and nutrition pumps, ensuring that nutrient solutions are administered at the prescribed rate.

2. **Infection prevention**: Artificial nutrition carries a high risk of infection, particularly for invasive devices such as parenteral nutrition catheters or gastrostomies. Caregivers

must be vigilant in ensuring **sterile handling**, taking care of insertion points and observing signs of infection, such as redness, discharge or fever.

3. **Monitoring the patient's general condition**: The caregiver must monitor **the patient's reactions** to artificial nutrition, in particular by observing signs of digestive discomfort (nausea, vomiting, diarrhea), variable tolerance of intake or signs of undernutrition (continued weight loss despite nutrition). By quickly reporting these anomalies to the medical team, he or she helps to adjust the care plan.

Moral and relational support

The relational and psychological aspects of the caregiver's work are just as important as the technical aspects. The caregiver is often the **daily point of reference** for patients and families. In this role, he or she must demonstrate great **empathy** and **active listening** skills, especially when decisions concerning artificial nutrition are fraught with consequences and difficult to accept.

1. **Accompanying the patient**: The caregiver is often the person who is closest to the patient on a day-to-day basis. When it comes to explaining artificial nutrition, reassuring patients about the procedure, or simply listening to their fears and frustrations, the caregiver acts as a **mediator** between the patient and the rest of the medical team. They can also be a reassuring presence for patients who feel isolated or anxious about the increasing dependence that artificial nutrition may involve.

2. **Supporting families**: Relatives can be particularly anxious about the introduction or continuation of artificial

nutrition. Caregivers can provide invaluable support to help them understand therapeutic choices, explain how devices work, and answer their questions about how artificial nutrition affects patient comfort. The caregiver's role is essential here, to **create a bond of trust** and provide clear, benevolent information.

Respecting patient choice

In situations where the patient is capable of expressing his or her wishes, the caregiver plays an important role in ensuring that **the patient's choices are respected**. He/she must ensure that the patient's wishes regarding artificial nutrition are respected, and that his/her dignity is preserved. If the patient refuses artificial nutrition or expresses the wish to stop the ,it caregiver must respect this decision, while ensuring that the patient enjoys optimum comfort.

In cases where the patient is no longer able to express herself/him, the role of the caregiver is to **facilitate communication between** the care team and the family, ensuring that the patient's choices, expressed through advance directives or the wishes of family and friends, are respected.

- Confidentiality and patient privacy

Confidentiality and respect for patient privacy are fundamental principles of medical and healthcare ethics. They ensure that a patient's personal and medical information remains strictly confidential and is shared only with those healthcare professionals directly involved in his or her care, and only to the extent necessary to provide appropriate care. These principles are essential to establishing and maintaining a **relationship of trust** between patient and caregiver, as they assure patients that their privacy will be protected and that sensitive information will not be disclosed without their consent.

In a medical environment where patients are often asked to share intimate, sometimes complex and potentially difficult information, respecting confidentiality is not only a legal obligation but also a moral imperative. This applies as much to medical aspects as to the personal aspects of the patient's life, whether it concerns his or her state of health, treatments, family history or social life.

The legal framework for confidentiality

The protection of patient confidentiality is governed by **national and international regulations**. In France, the **law on patients' rights** and the **Public Health Code** impose **absolute medical secrecy** on healthcare professionals. This legal framework is part of a long tradition that places the **protection of privacy** at the heart of medical ethics. What's more, the **General Data Protection Regulation (GDPR)**, applicable throughout the European Union, provides a strict framework for the use of personal data, including in the healthcare sector.

According to these laws, only those directly involved in the patient's care may have access to his or her medical data, and then only within the framework of that care. Any other disclosure, without the patient's explicit consent, is prohibited, except in exceptional cases defined by law (serious threats to public health, life-threatening emergencies, etc.).

Respect for confidentiality in daily practice

Respecting patient confidentiality involves a series of **daily practices** implemented by all medical and paramedical staff, including orderlies, nurses and doctors. All healthcare professionals, whatever their role, must ensure that patient privacy is respected in all aspects of care.

Restricted access to medical information

Only those involved in the patient's direct care have access to **medical records** or other confidential information. Caregivers should avoid discussing a patient's case in the presence of colleagues or third parties who are not directly involved in the patient's care. In addition, computer systems where medical data is stored must be protected by **passwords** and other security measures to ensure that only authorized persons can consult this information.

Discretion in discussions

Medical staff must exercise **discretion** when talking about a patient's health, especially in public areas of the hospital or in places where third parties might overhear. It is crucial not to discuss sensitive information in corridors, elevators or other communal areas where conversations could be overheard by uninvolved parties. Any discussion of a patient's condition should take place in a confidential environment, such as a closed office, to protect the patient's privacy.

Patient care

Privacy must also be guaranteed during direct patient care. When medical procedures or care are carried out, such as physical examinations or toilets, the patient's privacy must be preserved as far as possible. This means closing **the door**, **using curtains** in shared rooms, and **asking for the patient's consent** before performing intimate gestures. The patient must feel at ease and confident that his or her dignity is respected at all times.

Sharing information with the family

Respect for confidentiality also implies particular care in managing relations with the patient's family. Even if relatives wish to be informed about the patient's state of health, this can only be done with the **patient's explicit agreement**, unless the patient is incapable of expressing himself or herself, in which case decisions are made by legally designated persons or in accordance with the patient's advance directives. The patient has the right to choose what information can be shared with relatives, and to restrict access to certain details.

Specific challenges in the hospital environment

In the context of a hospital or care center, a number of challenges can arise with regard to **patient privacy**, especially in departments where care is provided collectively or in shared spaces. These situations call for heightened vigilance on the part of caregivers to ensure that the principles of confidentiality are maintained in an environment that is sometimes difficult to manage.

Shared rooms

In **shared rooms**, where several patients are grouped together, confidentiality can be compromised during medical discussions or care. It is therefore essential that caregivers :

- **Use separating curtains** to preserve patients' physical privacy during care.
- **Low-voiced** and avoid discussing overly sensitive subjects in the presence of other patients or visitors. If medical information needs to be shared, it is preferable to offer the patient a more confidential interview.

Medical consultations and discussions

It is common for medical discussions to take place with several caregivers around the patient's bed. However, these discussions must respect the patient's privacy by avoiding exposing sensitive information in front of other patients or uninvolved parties. Consultations can also be challenging, especially when sensitive subjects need to be discussed. In such situations, it's best to move the discussion to a confidential location, away from prying ears.

The caregiver's role in maintaining confidentiality

The **nursing auxiliary** plays a central role in respecting patient confidentiality on a daily basis. As a professional in close contact with the patient, the caregiver must ensure that practices strictly respect the patient's rights to confidentiality and privacy.

Respect for sensitive data and information

Caregivers must ensure that all information collected from patients, whether medical data or details of their personal lives, is kept strictly confidential. This information should only be shared with members of the medical team who are directly involved in the care, and never with other patients, visitors or staff not concerned. Caregivers must also be careful not to leave documents or files containing sensitive information lying around in places accessible to other people.

Discreet and respectful accompaniment

In their day-to-day support role, caregivers are often called upon to accompany patients in intimate situations, whether for personal care, grooming, or administering medication. They must ensure that **the** patient's **privacy is always preserved**, through respectful gestures, reassuring words and a caring attitude. In addition, they must be careful not to ask questions or broach sensitive subjects in front of others, unless the patient has given his or her consent to discuss them openly.

Confidentiality in file management

When handling medical records or documents containing personal information, caregivers must ensure that these documents are stored in secure locations that are not accessible to third parties.

The use of computer media to record or consult information must comply with current security protocols, such as locking screens when not in use.

The importance of ongoing training

Respecting patient confidentiality is a skill that requires regular, ongoing training. Nurses, like all healthcare professionals, need to be trained in **best practices** for managing confidentiality and protecting personal data. This training provides a reminder of the legal and ethical requirements for respecting privacy, and reinforces staff vigilance in the face of potentially risky situations.

3 The helping relationship: support beyond technical care

• Creating a relationship of trust with the patient

Creating a **relationship of trust with the patient** is one of the most fundamental and essential aspects of healthcare. This relationship of trust is based on elements such as active listening, empathy, transparency, respect and professional competence. It is the foundation on which all interaction between caregiver and patient rests, helping to establish a climate of security in which patients feel comfortable sharing their concerns, following medical recommendations and becoming actively involved in their own care.

Trust is crucial not only to improving the patient experience, but also to ensuring better **adherence to treatment**, **more accurate diagnosis**, and **effective communication** between caregiver and patient. Indeed, a patient who feels listened to and respected is more likely to collaborate, ask questions and express concerns that might otherwise go unnoticed.

The importance of active listening

Active listening is one of the first levers for establishing a relationship of trust with the patient. When the caregiver takes the time to really listen to what the patient has to say, without interruption or judgment, it creates a space where the patient feels heard and understood. Active listening is not just about paying attention to what is said, but also observing **non-verbal language** - facial expressions, tone of voice, and the patient's posture can reveal deep-seated emotions or concerns.

Active listening includes :

- **Taking time**: By letting patients express themselves without rushing them, caregivers show that they value their words. A patient who feels listened to confides more easily, facilitating a more accurate diagnosis and appropriate treatment.
- **Reformulate and ask questions**: To show that the caregiver has understood what the patient is saying, it's helpful to rephrase some of what the patient has said, and to ask open-ended questions that allow the points raised to be explored in greater depth. This shows that the caregiver is genuinely attentive to the patient's needs.
- **Being present**: Avoiding distractions, such as consulting a file in the middle of a conversation, helps create a climate of undivided attention and shows the patient that he or she is the center of attention.

Empathy: putting yourself in the patient's shoes

Empathy is an essential component of a trusting relationship. It enables the caregiver to understand what the patient is feeling, both physically and emotionally, without necessarily experiencing the same feelings. Showing empathy helps to create a deep human connection, which is indispensable in care, especially in situations where the patient may be feeling vulnerable, stressed or anxious.

To show empathy:

- **Acknowledging suffering or worry**: by using simple phrases such as "I understand how difficult this must be for you" or "It's normal to be worried in a situation like this", the caregiver validates the patient's emotions, which can have a calming effect.
- **Adapting your attitude**: Empathy is also expressed through gestures, such as a kind look, an open posture or a reassuring attitude. Sometimes, a simple, silent, comforting presence can be enough to build trust.
- **Personalize the exchange**: Patients appreciate being addressed in a **personalized** way, taking into account their experiences, fears and expectations. Asking questions about their daily lives, their family environment or their personal concerns creates a more authentic relationship.

Transparency and clear information

Transparency and **clear information** are essential for building trust, especially when important medical decisions are at stake. Patients must feel fully informed about their state of health, proposed treatments, potential side-effects and existing alternatives.

Care and treatment explained

Explaining care in a way that is **clear** and **adapted to the** patient's **level of understanding** is fundamental. Using complex medical terms without translating them can create a sense of distance and incomprehension. It is therefore essential to :

- **Simplify language**: using accessible, understandable terms helps patients to follow and appropriate explanations.
- **Clarifying the issues**: The caregiver must ensure that the patient understands the benefits, risks and alternatives of

proposed treatments. This includes an honest discussion of the possible side effects or consequences of certain medical decisions.

- **Inviting patients to ask questions**: Encouraging patients to ask questions shows that their opinions are taken into account and that their involvement is essential. They should never feel sidelined when it comes to making decisions about their health.

Respecting patient autonomy and choice

Respect for patient **autonomy** is another cornerstone of the relationship of trust. Patients must feel free to make choices concerning their treatment, after having been adequately informed. Although caregivers may have specific medical recommendations, the final choice rests with the patient. It is therefore important to :

- **Respecting patients' decisions**: Whether accepting or refusing treatment, caregivers must respect patients' decisions, even if they differ from medical recommendations. This respect for choices helps to build trust.
- **Involving patients in the decision-making process**: Patients must be **active participants in their own care**. Caregivers must actively involve them in discussions and decision-making, taking into account their values, priorities and personal wishes.

Professional competence as a guarantee of trust

Although the human aspect is paramount, the **professional competence** of caregivers remains a key factor in establishing a relationship of trust. Patients must be assured that the care they receive is of the highest quality and based on the best medical practices available. To achieve this, it is essential that :

- **Rigorous compliance with care protocols**: Compliance with **medical standards** and **care protocols** reassures patients of the quality and safety of the care they receive.
- **The caregiver shows himself to be competent and up-to-date**: Regular training, keeping abreast of the latest medical advances, and being able to answer the patient's questions accurately, reinforce confidence in the caregiver's ability to make the right decisions.

Time and continuity of care

Continuity of care is also an important factor in establishing and maintaining a relationship of trust. Patients feel more confident when they are cared for by a stable care team capable of understanding their medical history, anticipating their needs and responding consistently to their concerns.

The **time given** to patients, although sometimes limited in a hospital or clinical setting, is also crucial. When the caregiver takes the time to explain, listen and interact with the patient, it shows that the patient is the focus of attention. This attention, even when it takes the form of small gestures, reinforces the relationship of trust.

- Active listening to patients' anxieties and concerns

Active listening to **patients' anxieties** and **concerns** is a central element of the caregiver-patient relationship. When patients are faced with illness, complex treatments or an uncertain future, they may experience deep-seated emotions such as anxiety, fear or distress. Faced with these feelings, active listening becomes an indispensable skill for caregivers, as it helps to **reassure** patients, **reduce their stress**, and provide **emotional support** while reinforcing the quality of the therapeutic relationship.

Active listening involves not just hearing what the patient is saying, but **engaging fully** in the conversation, offering sincere attention and showing that he or she is understood and supported.

It's a practice that requires **empathy**, **patience** and **mental availability**.

The foundations of active listening

Active listening is characterized by attentive presence, validation of expressed emotions, and constructive interaction. It's not just about gathering medical information, but also **taking into account the** patient's **emotional experience**. In moments of anxiety, patients are not only looking for clinical answers, but above all for a space to **share their fears** and **feel that they are not alone**.

1. Create an environment conducive to discussion

To offer active listening, it is first essential to **create an environment** in which the patient feels comfortable talking about his or her anxieties. This means ensuring that the interview takes place in a calm, uninterrupted environment, where the patient can express themselves freely without feeling judged or pressured.

- **Ensuring an intimate, secure space**: Closing the door, keeping distractions at bay and avoiding interruptions help create an atmosphere conducive to confidence.
- **Adopt an open posture**: Turn towards the patient, look him or her in the eye, and show through posture and body language that you are fully available to him or her.

2. Validate the patient's emotions

One of the key components of active listening is the **validation of** the patient's **emotions**. When the patient expresses anxiety, it is crucial that the caregiver acknowledges his or her feelings and shows understanding. Rather than minimizing their fears or immediately looking for solutions, it's important to **give them the space** to express how they feel.

- **Acknowledging the legitimacy of worries**: Saying phrases like "I understand that this can be very worrying for you" or "It's normal to feel anxious in this situation" helps to show the patient that their emotions are legitimate and that you take them seriously.
- **Don't interrupt**: Letting the patient talk at his or her own pace, without interrupting, shows that you're available to listen, without trying to rush the conversation or impose immediate solutions.

3. Reformulate and clarify

To show that you've understood what the patient is saying, it's helpful to **rephrase** what he's saying or ask clarifying questions. This deepens the discussion and shows the patient that what he or she is saying has been taken into account.

- **Rephrase to validate understanding**: For example, if a patient expresses fears about a treatment, you can rephrase by saying: "If I understand correctly, you're worried about starting this treatment because you're afraid of the side effects. Is that correct?"
- **Ask open-ended questions**: To encourage the patient to develop his or her thoughts, open-ended questions, such as "Can you tell me more about what's worrying you?" or "What worries you most about this situation?", help to better pinpoint the origin of the anxiety.

Show empathy and compassion

Empathy is an essential component of active listening. It enables us to put ourselves in the patient's shoes and understand their feelings, without necessarily experiencing them ourselves. By offering empathic listening, the caregiver not only listens to the facts, but also to the emotions behind the words.

1. Adopt an empathetic attitude

Empathy is expressed not only in words, but also in tone of voice and body language. An empathetic attitude makes patients feel understood and supported, which can greatly reduce their anxiety.

- **Use a reassuring tone of voice**: Tone of voice plays a crucial role. A soft, reassuring tone can ease the patient's anxiety.
- **Expressing compassion**: Saying phrases like "I'm here for you" or "I understand this is a difficult situation" reinforces the idea that the patient is not alone in his or her fears.

2. Respect silence

Sometimes, patients may need **moments of silence** to reflect or collect their thoughts before continuing to talk about their concerns. Silence can be a powerful form of active listening, giving patients time to express themselves at their own pace. It's important not to fill these silences with words, but to respect them.

Helping patients identify their fears

Active listening not only gathers information, but also **helps patients better understand their** own anxieties. Sometimes, patients may have concerns that are diffuse or difficult to verbalize. By asking open-ended questions and offering attentive listening, the caregiver can help the patient clarify the source of his or her anxieties.

- **Identify sources of anxiety**: For example, a patient may say he's "anxious about hospitalization", but through active listening, he may reveal that his real fear is linked to isolation, pain or loss of control. Once this fear has been identified, the caregiver can provide specific, reassuring responses.

- **Helping to put emotions into words**: Some patients may find it difficult to verbalize their emotions. By rephrasing and asking targeted questions, the caregiver can help them express their feelings clearly, which can already bring some relief.

Offering appropriate, soothing responses

Once the patient's concerns and anxieties have been identified, it's important to offer **appropriate responses**, while taking care not to minimize their fears. Giving clear, reassuring information, without promising uncertain results, can help reduce anxiety.

1. Provide clear information

In many cases, **incomplete or misunderstood information** is at the root of patients' anxieties. After listening to the patient's concerns, the caregiver can provide precise explanations tailored to the patient's level of understanding. For example, if a patient is worried about a surgical procedure, it's helpful to explain every step of the process, risks and benefits, clearly and honestly.

2. Don't offer false assurances

Although the role of the caregiver is to allay concerns, it is essential to remain **authentic** and not give false assurances. Telling a patient that "everything will be all right" without being certain can create unrealistic expectations. It's more reassuring to say, "We'll do everything we can to make sure you're well looked after" or "I understand your concern, but we'll be there to support you every step of the way. »

Long-term monitoring and support

Active listening is not limited to a single moment in a patient's care. To establish a genuine **relationship of trust** and help the patient manage his or her anxieties on a long-term basis, it is important to **maintain active listening** throughout the treatment process.

- **Remaining available**: Patients need to know that they can express their anxieties at any time, and that their caregiver is ready to listen. This can take the form of regular follow-ups or more informal exchanges, where the patient is encouraged to talk freely about his or her concerns.
- **Adapting listening over time**: A patient's concerns may evolve over time. It's important to reassess anxieties on a regular basis, to provide ongoing, appropriate emotional support.

Chapter 11

Rehabilitation and reintegration of patients after hospitalization

1 Preparing for discharge: a key role for the caregiver

- Organizing home care: coordination with external services (home nursing, physiotherapy)

Organizing care at home is a key issue for patients who need ongoing medical care, but still wish to remain in their home environment. This often concerns patients in remission after hospitalization, the chronically ill, or the terminally ill. The aim of homecare is to ensure continuity of care, while enabling the patient to benefit from a more intimate and soothing environment. For this care to be optimal, **effective coordination** with **external services** such as home nursing, physiotherapy and other healthcare professionals is essential. This organization must be rigorous, fluid and adapted to the specific needs of each patient.

Assessing the patient's needs

The first step in organizing care at home is to **draw up a complete assessment of the patient's needs**. This assessment should be carried out before discharge from hospital, or in consultation with the medical team if the patient is already at home. It involves assessing :

- Specific medical needs, such as the administration of medication, post-operative care or monitoring of a chronic pathology;
- **Nursing** needs, for example, for dressings, catheter monitoring, infusion management or artificial nutrition;
- **Rehabilitation** needs, such as physiotherapy or occupational therapy, to maintain or restore mobility and autonomy;
- The need for **technical aids**, such as medical devices (wheelchairs, medical beds, etc.) that facilitate the patient's daily life;
- **Psychosocial** aspects, such as the psychological and moral support required by patients and their families.

This assessment helps to build a **personalized care plan**, centered on the patient's needs and preferences. Once this assessment has been carried out, it is essential to establish seamless coordination between the various external parties involved.

Coordination with home nursing care

Homecare nurses are often the first external professionals involved in homecare, particularly for technical or supervisory care. Their role is crucial in managing day-to-day health care, and their coordination with the attending physician or hospital must be flawless.

Transmission of medical information

One of the first aspects of coordination is the **transmission of medical information** between the hospital (or attending physician) and the homecare team. This includes:

- Specific **medical prescriptions,** with clear instructions on the treatments to be administered;
- An **account of hospital treatment** or a summary of current treatments;
- Detailed instructions for medical devices to be monitored or handled (probes, catheters, complex dressings, etc.).

This information needs to be **regularly updated** and clearly communicated, to avoid mismanagement. Homecare nurses must be able to consult doctors in case of doubt or need to adjust treatment.

Nursing care organization

Home care must be organized according to a **precise schedule**, with interventions tailored to the patient's needs. This may include:

- **Regular visits** for injections, infusion management or technical care;

335

- **More frequent visits** in critical phases, such as after surgery or when a chronic pathology is decompensating;
- **Monitoring visits** to ensure that the patient's health is progressing well, and to adjust care if necessary.

The home care nurse also plays a key role in **clinical monitoring**, detecting the first signs of complications (infections, deterioration in general condition) and alerting the medical team if necessary.

Coordination with physiotherapy and rehabilitation

In many cases, home care includes **physiotherapy** or **occupational therapy sessions** to help the patient regain or maintain a degree of mobility and autonomy. Coordination with these professionals is crucial to ensure effective rehabilitation.

Transmission of rehabilitation goals

The attending physician or rehabilitation physician must draw up a **detailed rehabilitation plan**, specifying the objectives to be achieved, the exercises recommended and the points to be monitored. These objectives should be passed on to the **home physiotherapists**, who will adapt their intervention according to the patient's progress.

Regular communication between the physiotherapist and the medical team is essential to adjust the treatment. For example, if a patient recovers faster than expected or, on the contrary, if complications arise, the rehabilitation plan will need to be adjusted accordingly.

Organization of rehabilitation sessions

Physiotherapy sessions should be planned on a regular basis, taking into account **the patient's availability and** physical capabilities. Sessions can be intensified after hospitalization or during periods of active rehabilitation, then reduced to maintenance visits once the goal of recovery has been achieved.

Coordination with other external services

In addition to nursing care and physiotherapy, other services can be mobilized to provide comprehensive care at home. These services may include :

- **Care assistants** to help with washing, eating and daily mobility;
- **Nutrition services** for patients receiving enteral or parenteral nutrition;
- **Psychologists** for emotional support, particularly for patients in palliative care or facing chronic disabling illnesses;
- **Occupational therapists** to adapt the home environment to the patient's functional abilities (installation of grab bars, adaptation of furniture).

These professionals work in coordination with the home care nurse and the doctor to adapt daily care.

Management of technical and logistical aids

Home care organization also includes the **logistical management of medical devices** and **supplies needed** for care. This may include:

- Installation of **medical beds**, wheelchairs, walkers or other mobility aids;
- Regular delivery of **medical supplies** such as dressings, catheters and infusions;
- Installation of **remote monitoring** systems for patients requiring continuous monitoring of vital parameters.

The caregiver in charge of organization must ensure that equipment is delivered on time and that devices are installed correctly to avoid any interruption in care.

The role of family and caregivers

Family and **caregivers** play an essential role in the organization of homecare. They must be integrated into the coordination process, as they will often be the first point of contact for healthcare professionals, and the ones who will look after the patient's day-to-day well-being.

Caregiver training

To facilitate home care, **family caregivers** need to be trained in certain tasks, such as :

- Use of simple medical devices (probes, nutrition pumps);
- Monitoring warning signs that should be reported to caregivers;
- Participation in hygiene care or assistance with daily tasks.

It's important that family caregivers feel **accompanied** and **supported**, as the burden of care can be heavy. Home carers must also take care not to overburden families, and to offer them **respite solutions** if necessary.

Monitoring and adjusting care plans

Homecare needs to be **evaluated regularly** to adjust the care plan to the patient's changing state of health. This requires fluid communication between :

- The attending physician ;
- Home care nurses ;
- Physiotherapists and other healthcare professionals.

This assessment enables us to decide whether the patient requires **further care**, whether he or she can move on to less intensive follow-up, or whether emergency interventions are necessary in the event of complications.

- The caregiver's role in educating the patient about continuing care at home (stoma management, gastric tube)

The caregiver's role in educating the patient about continuing care at home is fundamental to ensuring continuity of care and promoting patient autonomy, particularly in complex situations such as **ostomy** or **gastric tube** management. The caregiver is often the patient's first point of contact when it comes to daily and technical care. As such, they play a key role not only in initial hospital care, but also in supporting and educating patients to enable them to manage their medical devices effectively once they return home.

This education is essential to ensure that patients can **continue their care safely**, minimize the risk of complications and improve their quality of life. By offering clear, practical advice tailored to the patient's level of understanding, the caregiver contributes directly to empowering the patient and reducing re-hospitalization.

The importance of patient education

Patient education on home care management, such as ostomies or gastric tubes, has several key objectives:

- **Reinforce** patients' **autonomy** by enabling them to take responsibility for part of their daily care.
- **Reduce complications** arising from improper handling or maintenance of medical devices.
- **Ease** patient and family **concerns** about managing complex technical care.
- **Improve** patients' **quality of life** by giving them the tools they need to live more serenely with their device.

With their hands-on approach and direct contact with the patient, caregivers are ideally placed to meet these objectives.

Ostomy management education

The management of **ostomies**, whether colostomies, ileostomies or urostomies, is often a source of stress and anxiety for patients. These devices, although life-saving, require a major adjustment in daily life, both physically and psychologically.

Learning to handle the stoma

The caregiver must teach the patient the basics of **stoma care and handling**. This includes specific technical gestures, but also practical advice on how to integrate this care into daily life.

1. **Changing the pouch**: The patient must learn to change the ostomy pouch independently. The caregiver demonstrates how to remove the old pouch, properly clean the skin around the stoma, apply a skin protector if necessary, and safely reposition a new pouch.

2. **Preventing skin irritation**: The skin around the stoma is sensitive and prone to irritation. The caregiver explains how to **prevent redness** and infection, making sure the area is always clean and dry, and checking that the pouch fits properly to prevent leakage. They can also recommend suitable skin care products.

3. **Leak and odor management**: The caregiver must also reassure the patient about **leak** and **odor** management. This can include advice on the choice of suitable bags, the use of odor filters, and tips on how to prevent accidents, for example by avoiding overfilling the bag or emptying it regularly.

Encouraging autonomy

Over time, the caregiver must encourage the patient to take responsibility for managing his or her stoma independently. This involves :

- **Gradually allow patients to handle** the stoma **themselves**, under supervision, until they feel confident enough to manage care without assistance.
- **Reassure and encourage** patients about their abilities, as ostomy management can generate initial fears. The caregiver plays a central role in providing moral support and dispelling doubts.

Answering patients' questions

Patients and their families may have many questions about their stoma, such as what type of food to eat, how to get around or what precautions to take when playing sports. The caregiver must provide clear, practical answers, taking into account the specific needs of each patient.

Education on gastric tube management

Gastric tubes, whether nasogastric or gastrostomy (PEG), also require rigorous home care. These devices are used for enteral feeding and, in some cases, to evacuate gastric secretions. Caregivers play an essential role in teaching patients how to **use** these devices, and the **precautions** to be taken to avoid complications.

Sensor maintenance

The caregiver must teach the patient (or family) how to **care for the catheter** correctly, to avoid blockages or infections.

1. **Rinsing the tube**: After each use, the gastric tube must be **rinsed** to prevent food residues from accumulating and clogging the tube. The caregiver demonstrates how to use sterile water to rinse the tube and ensure it remains functional.

2. **Insertion site monitoring**: In the case of gastrostomy (PEG), the site where the tube is inserted into the stomach

341

can be prone to infection or irritation. The caregiver teaches how to **clean the site** daily with appropriate solutions, and how to spot signs of infection such as redness, pain or discharge.

Nutrient administration

The caregiver must also explain how to **administer nutrients** via the tube. This step includes several specific sub-tasks that require clear and appropriate training.

1. **Preparing nutrition**: Patients and their families need to learn how to prepare **nutrient solutions** or use ready-to-use pouches, ensuring that they are at the right temperature and contain the elements prescribed by the doctor.

2. **Using pump or gravity**: Some patients use a **nutrition pump** to administer nutrients continuously, while others may use **gravity administration**. The caregiver demonstrates how to set up the pump, adjust the flow rate, and check that nutrition is being delivered correctly. He or she must also teach how to watch for signs of **poor tolerance** (nausea, vomiting, diarrhea).

Preventing and managing complications

Gastric tubes can lead to **complications** such as infections, obstructions or displacement of the tube. The caregiver trains the patient or family to **identify warning signs**:

*   **Abdominal pain** or suspicious discharge around the gastrostomy site;

- **Difficulty administering nutrition**, a sign that the tube may be obstructed;
- **Irritation or redness** around the nose or PEG site;
- **Accidental displacement or removal of the probe**, requiring rapid intervention.

Helping patients make the transition home

Patient support is not limited to technical procedures. It also includes **psychological and practical** support to help them deal with the emotional and logistical aspects of managing these medical devices.

Reassurance and confidence-building

Patients may feel anxious about managing their stoma or catheter at home on their own. The caregiver plays a key role in **reassuring the patient** of his or her ability to manage this care. By providing encouragement and answering any questions, the caregiver reinforces the **patient's** self-confidence and competence.

Involving family and friends

In some cases, the management of care in the home may rest partly on the patient's relatives. The caregiver must therefore ensure that these relatives are also trained in technical gestures, and that they feel comfortable assisting the patient in this care. **Clear training** is essential to ensure that caregivers know how to react in the event of a problem.

Regular monitoring and reassessment

Education does not end when the patient is discharged from hospital. The caregiver must ensure that the patient receives

regular follow-up to check that care at home is going well, and to answer any questions that may emerge over time. This may involve **home visits** or remote consultations to adjust care as the situation evolves.

2 Functional rehabilitation after surgery or heavy treatment

- Supporting the patient's post-operative recovery (early mobilization, breathing exercises)

Supporting patients in their **post-operative recovery** is a crucial step in optimizing convalescence, preventing complications and enabling them to return to independence as quickly as possible. After surgery, whether minor or major, the body undergoes a phase of readjustment that requires attentive support from the caregivers. Caregivers play a central role in this process, particularly by encouraging **early mobilization** and supervising **breathing exercises**. These actions, although often perceived as simple post-operative measures, have a profound impact on recovery and the prevention of complications such as pulmonary infections or venous thrombosis.

Early mobilization: a key factor in avoiding complications

Early mobilization is one of the most important aspects of post-operative recovery. Encouraging the patient to get up and moving as soon as possible after surgery helps to limit complications associated with immobility, such as **deep vein thrombosis (DVT)**, **respiratory infections**, **pressure sores** and muscle loss.

Objectives of early mobilization

The benefits of early mobilization are manifold:

1. **Prevention of thromboembolic complications**: By mobilizing muscles, even slightly, blood flow is activated,

reducing the risk of clots forming in deep veins. Thrombosis, if not prevented, can lead to serious pulmonary embolism.

2. **Maintaining muscle function**: Prolonged immobility leads to rapid loss of muscle mass, making long-term rehabilitation more difficult. Early mobilization helps maintain muscle strength and avoid atrophy.

3. **Improved circulation**: Exercise activates blood and lymph circulation, helping to prevent oedema, promote healing and accelerate overall recovery.

4. **Pressure sore prevention**: Immobilized patients are at risk of developing pressure sores. By encouraging regular, even light movements, the risk of prolonged pressure on certain areas of the body is reduced.

The caregiver's role in mobilization

The nursing auxiliary is in the front line, encouraging and assisting the patient in his or her first mobilizations. This is a gradual process that must be carried out with care, taking into account post-operative pain, surgical restrictions and the patient's general condition.

1. **Get up as soon as possible**: According to medical recommendations, caregivers encourage patients to sit on the edge of the bed in the first few hours after surgery, subject to approval by the surgeon or medical team. This will help to restore balance and promote gradual muscular recovery.

2. **Help with walking**: When it's possible for the patient to get up, the caregiver provides physical support by accompanying him/her as he/she takes his/her first steps, whether in the room or in the hospital corridor. This gradual approach helps the patient gradually regain

345

confidence in his or her physical abilities, while avoiding excessive bed rest.

3. **Monitoring and encouragement**: It's essential for the caregiver to monitor **the patient's reactions**, such as dizziness, signs of intense fatigue, or unusual pain. While listening carefully, he or she must encourage the patient to gently push back his or her limits, without forcing him or her.

4. **Correct positioning**: The caregiver ensures that the patient is in a seated or semi-seated position when in bed, and changes position regularly to avoid pressure points that can cause pressure sores.

Breathing exercises: preventing pulmonary complications

Breathing exercises are another pillar of post-operative recovery, particularly after abdominal or thoracic surgery, or when general anesthesia has been used. Post-operative immobility, pain and sedation can affect respiratory capacity, favoring the development of pulmonary complications such as **atelectasis** or **pneumonia**. Encouraging the patient to perform breathing exercises helps improve pulmonary ventilation and maintain a good level of oxygenation.

Objectives of breathing exercises

1. **Reopening the pulmonary alveoli**: After general anesthesia, certain areas of the lungs may partially close, reducing breathing capacity. Breathing exercises help reopen the alveoli, improving oxygenation and reducing the risk of atelectasis.

2. **Prevention of lung infections**: By stimulating deep breathing, exercises help to clear secretions from the

346

respiratory tract, preventing them from stagnating and reducing the risk of infections such as pneumonia.

3. **Pain reduction**: Deep, controlled breathing can also help manage post-operative pain by allowing the patient to relax and avoid painful shallow breathing.

The caregiver's role in breathing exercises

The caregiver plays a fundamental role in supporting the patient's breathing exercises, explaining how to perform them correctly and motivating him or her to practice them regularly.

1. **Encourage deep breathing**: As soon as the patient is awake after surgery, the caregiver encourages him or her to take **deep breaths** by inflating the abdomen, then exhaling slowly. This simple exercise can be repeated several times an hour.

2. **Use of an incentive spirometer**: If an **incentive** spirometer is prescribed, the caregiver shows the patient how to use it correctly. This device helps visualize breathing amplitude and encourages the patient to take deep breaths to maintain good lung function. The caregiver ensures that the patient uses it regularly and under the right conditions.

3. **Controlled coughing**: The caregiver also teaches the patient how to practice **controlled coughing** to expel bronchial secretions. This involves taking a deep breath, holding it for a few seconds, then gently expelling the air by coughing. This exercise can be particularly useful after abdominal or thoracic surgery, and the caregiver ensures that the patient supports the operated area with his or her hands or a pillow to avoid pain during coughing.

Managing pain and encouraging activity

Pain is a factor that can limit mobilization and breathing exercises. It is therefore essential that the caregiver is attentive to the patient's **pain management**, so that the patient is able to move and breathe without undue discomfort.

Pain monitoring and assessment

The caregiver regularly assesses the intensity of the patient's pain using specific scales (numerical scale, visual analog scale), and ensures that the **prescribed analgesics** are optimally administered before key moments of mobilization or breathing exercises.

Encouragement despite pain

It's important to emphasize that, although post-operative pain is unavoidable in some cases, it must not prevent the patient from performing **activities essential** to recovery. The caregiver, while respecting the patient's limitations, must explain that moving and breathing deeply, even in the presence of moderate pain, is crucial to avoid more serious complications.

Regular monitoring and reassessment

Finally, the caregiver is responsible for **regularly monitoring the patient's progress**. They must monitor the progress of mobilization and breathing exercises, and adjust their approach according to the patient's needs and condition. This involves :

- Note the progress made in terms of mobility and breathing;
- Report any complications or difficulties encountered (e.g. signs of respiratory decompensation or pain that prevents exercise) to the medical team;

- Continue to motivate the patient, even after the first critical days, so that efforts are maintained.

- The importance of nutrition in the rehabilitation process

Nutrition plays a fundamental role in the **rehabilitation process** following illness, surgery or trauma. Proper nutrition not only promotes healing, but also supports muscle recovery, strengthens the immune system and improves the patient's quality of life. In rehabilitation, whether in the post-operative phase or in the long-term management of a chronic disease, nutrition is much more than just energy support: it becomes an essential therapeutic lever.

The role of nutrition in healing and recovery

After surgery or injury, the body requires optimal nutritional intake to ensure **effective healing** and **repair of** damaged **tissue**. Healing is a complex process that mobilizes significant resources, and without sufficient **nutrient** intake, this process can be slowed down, increasing the risk of complications.

Proteins: essential elements for tissue repair

Proteins play a central role in **tissue reconstruction** and the **synthesis of enzymes** required for healing. They provide essential amino acids for the production of collagen, the key protein in the formation of scar tissue. In patients undergoing rehabilitation, insufficient protein intake can compromise wound healing, prolong hospitalization and increase the risk of infection.

Patients who have undergone surgery or injury should therefore be given a diet rich in **high-quality proteins**, such as lean meat, fish, eggs and dairy products. In some cases, protein-rich nutritional supplements may be recommended, particularly for elderly or malnourished patients, who often have increased protein requirements.

Micronutrients and wound healing

In addition to proteins, specific **micronutrients** are also essential for wound healing:

- **Zinc** is involved in cell regeneration and wound healing.
- **Vitamin C** is crucial for collagen synthesis and has antioxidant properties that help protect tissues undergoing repair.
- **Iron** contributes to tissue oxygenation by promoting the production of red blood cells, essential for transporting oxygen to damaged areas.

A lack of these nutrients can lead to poor healing, infections and delayed rehabilitation.

Nutrition and maintaining muscle mass

One of the main aims of rehabilitation, especially after long-term hospitalization or immobilization, is to prevent **muscle loss** and **restore strength**. **Sarcopenia**, i.e. loss of muscle mass, is common in patients confined to bed or weakened by illness. Without appropriate nutrition, this muscle loss can compromise physical rehabilitation, making recovery more difficult and delaying the return to independence.

Protein and muscle rehabilitation

Protein is once again a central pillar in supporting muscle rehabilitation. The supply of essential amino acids, particularly **leucine**, is particularly important in stimulating protein synthesis and promoting muscle rebuilding. In the post-operative phase or after prolonged immobilization, adequate protein intake helps to limit muscle degradation and accelerate recovery.

The importance of calories

In addition to protein, adequate caloric intake is essential to provide the energy needed for muscle rehabilitation. Patients who don't consume enough calories to meet their metabolic needs run an increased risk of muscle loss and weakness. This can prolong their recovery time and make physical rehabilitation more difficult. **Complex carbohydrates** and **healthy fats** must therefore form an integral part of the diet to ensure a balanced energy intake.

Boosting the immune system

Adequate nutrition is also essential for strengthening the **immune system**, which is often weakened after surgery or illness. A healthy immune system helps to fight infection and reduce the risk of complications such as hospital-acquired infections and post-operative complications.

The role of nutrients in immunity

Certain vitamins and minerals play a direct role in the functioning of the immune system. For example:

- **Vitamin A** helps maintain the integrity of mucous membranes and skin, physical barriers against infection.
- **Vitamin D** is involved in regulating the immune response, and a deficiency can make the patient more vulnerable to infection.
- **Zinc** and **selenium** contribute to the proper functioning of immune cells, particularly lymphocytes, which play a key role in defending against infection.

By maintaining an optimal intake of these micronutrients, patients can benefit from enhanced immune protection during rehabilitation.

Preventing nutritional complications

Rehabilitation patients are often exposed to **nutritional complications**, such as undernutrition, due to reduced appetite, post-operative pain, or fatigue. **Undernutrition** can not only slow recovery, but also worsen the patient's overall health, increasing the risk of post-operative complications and hospital readmissions.

Nutritional screening and monitoring

It is crucial that healthcare professionals, including **nursing aides**, are alert to signs of undernutrition in rehabilitation patients. Involuntary weight loss, reduced appetite or difficulty in eating should be reported promptly, so that nutritional intake can be adjusted. Oral **nutritional supplements**, in the form of protein- and calorie-enriched drinks, may be necessary to make up for deficiencies and prevent undernutrition.

Adapting diets to specific needs

In some cases, rehabilitation patients may require specific diets depending on their pathology or surgery. For example:

- After **digestive surgery**, it may be necessary to adapt the texture of food or limit certain types of food to avoid irritation of the digestive tract.
- Patients with **kidney disease** may need a diet low in protein, sodium or potassium.
- Diabetic patients need to monitor their carbohydrate intake to maintain optimal glycemic control.

In these situations, the caregiver plays an important role in ensuring that the prescribed diet is adhered to, and in helping to educate the patient about any necessary dietary adjustments.

Nutrition-related psychological support

The psychological impact of nutrition in rehabilitation should not be underestimated. For many patients, food is not only a source of energy, but also an element of comfort and pleasure. After illness or surgery, some patients may find it difficult to re-establish a positive relationship with food, not least because of dietary restrictions or fear of eating certain foods.

Caregivers, in collaboration with **dieticians**, can play a key role in encouraging patients to take a positive approach to nutrition, explaining the importance of food intake for recovery and finding solutions to make meals more enjoyable and suited to their tastes.

3 Social and professional reintegration of gastroenterology patients

• Helping patients resume their daily and professional lives
Supporting patients as they resume their daily and professional lives is a decisive phase in the healing and rehabilitation process. After illness, hospitalization or surgery, the return to normality can be a complex challenge. It's not just a question of physical recovery: reintegration into daily and professional life also requires psychological, social and often practical adaptation. Caregivers, particularly nursing assistants, have a key role to play in this process. They help patients gradually regain their autonomy, supporting them at every stage of their return to active life.

The importance of progressive rehabilitation

Progressive rehabilitation is a fundamental principle in facilitating the successful resumption of daily and professional activities. It is essential to take into account the patient's physical and psychological state, as well as any functional limitations, to enable him or her to gradually return to his or her own pace of life, without risking relapse or overload.

Resuming physical and daily activities

After a long period of rest or convalescence, it can be difficult for the patient to resume domestic activities, such as household chores, getting around or managing family life. **Loss of mobility,** post-operative **fatigue** or the after-effects of the disease may limit the patient's ability to reintegrate into daily life.

The role of caregivers is to guide the patient towards a **gradual resumption of physical activity** according to his or her abilities and medical recommendations. This includes :

- **Plan adapted activities**: Encourage the patient to resume simple daily activities, such as getting up regularly, walking or performing light domestic tasks. These activities not only promote physical recovery, but also a sense of autonomy and self-confidence.
- **Supporting fatigue management**: Caregivers need to help patients balance effort and rest. Excessive fatigue can be discouraging and counterproductive, while insufficient activity can slow recovery.
- **Adapting the home if necessary**: In some cases, it may be necessary to make **adjustments** to the patient's living environment, such as installing grab bars or organizing the space to minimize physical effort and ensure safety.

Psychological preparation for returning to work

Psychologically, the return to a normal life can be **a** source of **stress, anxiety** and **lack of** self-confidence, especially if the illness or operation was traumatic or accompanied by significant limitations. Many patients express fears about their ability to resume their former pace of life, or to resume their professional responsibilities, especially if they have been absent for long periods.

Caregivers play a crucial role in providing **emotional support** to patients:

- **Encouragement and reassurance**: Caregivers need to listen to the patient's concerns and offer regular encouragement. They can also reassure them that the

354

rehabilitation process takes time, and that it's normal to encounter obstacles along the way.

- **Supporting stress management**: For some patients, the anxiety associated with resuming activities can be intense. The caregiver can help by suggesting relaxation exercises, or referring the patient to **psychological support** if necessary.

A gradual return to professional life

Returning to work after a long period of illness or convalescence can be an even greater challenge. **Reintegration into the world of work** requires both physical and psychological preparation, as well as coordination with employers and occupational health services to ensure a smooth transition.

Adapting the return to work

In many cases, a **gradual return** to work is recommended. It is important to prepare for this return by taking into account the patient's ability to assume his or her former responsibilities without risking compromising his or her health.

1. **Part-time therapy**: For patients who cannot immediately return to work on a full-time basis, **part-time therapy** is often introduced. This enables the patient to return to work slowly, with reduced working hours, while continuing to benefit from medical supervision.

2. **Workstation adjustments**: Depending on the nature of the patient's job, specific **adjustments may** be required, such as reducing physical tasks, lightening responsibilities or modifying the work environment. Caregivers, in collaboration with ergonomists and the occupational physician, can help identify these needs and prepare the necessary adjustments.

3. **Communication with the employer**: Caregivers can advise the patient to engage in **open communication** with his or her employer to define the terms of return. This communication is essential to avoid the pressure of a hasty return, and to establish a realistic plan for resuming work.

Building confidence and motivation

Returning to work can raise **doubts** in patients, who often wonder whether they'll be able to get back to their usual pace, assume their responsibilities or continue to perform at their best. The caregiver's job is to **reinforce the** patient's self-confidence:

- **Valuing progress**: It's important to remind patients of the steps they have already successfully taken, to show them that gradual reintegration into working life is a logical step in their rehabilitation process.
- **Setting achievable goals**: Helping patients set **realistic goals** for their return to work helps prevent burnout and disappointment, and maintains a sense of continuous progress.

Managing fatigue and physical limitations

After illness or surgery, **fatigue** may persist for a long time, limiting the patient's ability to work at full capacity. It's crucial that patients learn to manage this fatigue, by taking time out to rest and adapting their work rhythm.

Caregivers can :

- **Teaching time and energy management**: Knowing how to plan tasks according to energy levels enables patients to remain productive without burning out. This includes taking regular breaks and adjusting schedules if necessary.
- **Preventing overwork**: Patients need to be made aware of the signs of overwork, such as persistent fatigue, pain or

loss of concentration, and not hesitate to adjust their schedules or ask for help if necessary.

Medical follow-up and adjustments

The return to everyday life and work should not be rushed. **Regular medical follow-up** is essential to adjust the reintegration plan in line with changes in the patient's health. The attending physician, in collaboration with the care team, must assess the patient's progress and decide whether adjustments are necessary.

Post-operative or post-illness follow-up

Depending on the nature of the pathology or operation, the patient may require **regular consultations** to monitor recovery, particularly in the case of chronic illness or major surgery. These consultations enable us to assess the patient's general condition, adapt treatments or care, and ensure that resumption of activities takes place without complications.

Reassessment of functional capabilities

Regular check-ups may also be necessary to **reassess the** patient's **physical capabilities** and adjust recommendations. These include mobility tests, muscle strength tests, or general health check-ups, to assess whether the patient can gradually increase his or her level of activity.

Accompanying loved ones and providing psychological support

The **patient's family and friends** play an important role in the patient's return to everyday life and work. They are often the patient's primary psychological and practical support, but can also be affected by the illness or convalescence. Caregivers must ensure that their loved ones are included in the rehabilitation process.

Emotional support and information

Relatives may need **advice** and **support** to understand the patient's needs and help him or her appropriately. Their involvement is invaluable in promoting reintegration, but they also need to be informed about the patient's limitations and ways of supporting him/her without overprotecting or overburdening him/her.

Preventing caregiver burnout

Caregiver support is also essential to avoid caregiver burnout. They need to be encouraged to take care of themselves, while offering assistance in reintegrating the patient into daily life. Caregivers can also refer families to **support resources** or home help services to lighten their load.

• Tips for managing food and activities after hospitalization
After hospitalization, the management of food and activities plays a crucial role in the patient's recovery and reintegration into daily life. Care doesn't stop when you leave hospital: that's when a delicate period begins in which diet and activities must be **gradually adapted to** ensure optimal healing, prevent complications and regain the energy needed to resume normal activities. Whether hospitalization is due to an acute illness, surgery or an exacerbation of a chronic disease, patients need **tailored advice** to manage this transition smoothly. Here are a few recommendations to guide patients in managing their diet and activities after hospitalization.

Adapting your diet to support recovery

Post-hospitalization nutrition is essential to support **recovery**, promote **healing** and restore energy. After hospitalization, the body can be weakened, and it needs the right nutritional intake to rebuild. The diet must therefore be balanced, rich in essential nutrients, and adapted to the patient's digestive capacities, which may be impaired.

Promoting a nutrient-rich diet

The priority is to provide the **nutrients** needed for recovery:

- **Protein**: Essential for tissue repair and muscle recovery. Lean protein sources, such as eggs, fish, poultry, tofu or legumes, should be preferred. If the patient has increased needs (e.g. after surgery), protein-rich **nutritional supplements** may be considered.
- **Vitamins and minerals**: Micronutrients such as **vitamin C**, essential for healing, **zinc** for the immune system, and **iron** to combat anemia, must be provided by a varied diet. Fresh fruit and vegetables, as well as iron-rich foods such as spinach and lean red meat, should be consumed regularly.
- **Hydration**: Good **hydration** is crucial, especially after hospitalization. Water, herbal teas and broths are preferred to avoid dehydration, which can occur rapidly after illness or surgery.

Adapting food to specific needs

Some patients may have specific dietary requirements, depending on the nature of their hospitalization or their state of health:

- **Light diet** after abdominal surgery: For patients who have undergone digestive surgery, an **easy-to-digest diet** is recommended, such as soups, compotes or purées, before gradually reintroducing more solid foods. This helps to protect the digestive system while ensuring adequate nutritional intake.
- **Meal splitting**: After hospitalization, appetite and digestive capacity may be reduced. It is therefore

359

advisable to **divide meals into** several small portions throughout the day, to avoid feelings of heaviness and ensure a continuous supply of energy.

- **Avoid irritating foods**: In some cases, foods can be irritating or difficult to digest after hospitalization, especially for patients with digestive diseases. We recommend avoiding fatty, spicy or acidic foods, as well as carbonated beverages, to prevent digestive discomfort.

Monitor weight regain or undernutrition

After hospitalization, some patients may have lost weight involuntarily or show signs of **undernutrition**. It is important to monitor the patient's weight and nutritional status, particularly in the case of the elderly or those with increased energy requirements. If diet alone is not sufficient to meet nutritional needs, **food supplements** can be introduced, always in consultation with a dietician or healthcare professional.

Gradually resume physical activity

After hospitalization, **resumption of physical activity** should be gradual and adapted to the patient's state of health. Prolonged immobility during hospitalization can lead to **muscle loss**, reduced mobility and general fatigue. It is therefore crucial to resume physical activity slowly, respecting the body's capabilities and taking into account medical recommendations.

Early mobilization and gentle activities

As soon as they leave hospital, patients should be encouraged to get moving, but without rushing. **Gentle activities** such as walking are an excellent way of gradually regaining mobility and preventing complications associated with immobility, such as venous thrombosis or bedsores.

- **Walking**: We recommend starting with **short strolls** several times a day, gradually increasing duration and distance according to the patient's tolerance. Walking helps stimulate blood circulation, strengthens muscles and improves breathing.

- **Breathing exercises**: After surgery, particularly abdominal or thoracic surgery, breathing exercises are essential to **prevent pulmonary complications**. Patients should be encouraged to practice regular deep breathing, and to use an incentive spirometer if prescribed.
- **Avoid sudden exertion**: It's important to remind patients to avoid sudden or intense physical exertion, especially after surgery. Lifting heavy objects, running or resuming sporting activities too soon can lead to complications or a recurrence of symptoms.

Plan a gradual increase in activity

The return to normal physical activity, including sports, should be a gradual process. Depending on the patient's state of health and the type of operation or illness, the plan for resuming physical activity will be adjusted accordingly.

- **Gradually strengthen muscles**: After a long period of hospitalization or rest, muscles can become weakened. **Gentle muscle-strengthening** exercises are recommended, such as stretching, sheathing or the use of light resistance elastics.
- **Schedule rehabilitation exercises**: For some patients, **functional rehabilitation** under the supervision of a physiotherapist may be necessary to restore mobility and strength after surgery or trauma. These targeted, progressive exercises help prevent joint stiffness and restore the patient's physical capabilities.

Manage fatigue and listen to your body

One of the most delicate aspects of the post-hospitalization period is **managing fatigue**. Fatigue can persist long after illness or surgery, and it is essential that patients learn to recognize their limitations and adapt their activities accordingly.

Plan regular rest periods

Post-operative or post-illness fatigue is normal, but needs to be carefully managed. Patients are advised to alternate between **periods of activity** and **rest** to avoid physical exhaustion. Patients should be encouraged to listen to their bodies and rest as soon as they experience significant fatigue.

Avoid returning to a normal rhythm too quickly

It's tempting for some patients to want to **return quickly to their** usual **activities**, or even their jobs, after hospitalization. However, this rush can be counter-productive, leading to relapses or slowing down the healing process. Patients should be encouraged to respect the pace of recovery that their bodies dictate, avoiding **overzealousness**.

Follow medical recommendations

Each patient is unique, and resumption of activities should be based on the doctor's **specific recommendations**. In some cases, regular check-ups are necessary to assess the progress of recovery and adjust activities according to the results.

Psychological and social support after hospitalization

The post-hospitalization period can also be **psychologically** challenging. Feelings of vulnerability, anxiety about resuming activities or fear of complications are common among patients, especially after a long convalescence.

Listening and moral support

Caregivers, but also family and friends, play a key role in providing **psychological support** to patients after hospitalization. It's essential to listen attentively, reassure them of their ability to recover, and remind them that rehabilitation is a process that takes time.

Encouraging socialization

Resuming **light social activities** is just as important as resuming physical activity. Contact with friends and family, or participation in gentle social activities, can help **reduce stress** and maintain a positive state of mind, essential for recovery.

Chapter 12

Caring for patients at the end of life in gastroenterology

1 The role of palliative care in gastroenterology

- When digestive disease becomes incurable: the role of palliative care

When **digestive disease becomes incurable**, care priorities shift from cure to patient **comfort, symptom relief** and **quality of life**. This is where **palliative care** comes in, an essential approach to supporting patients with advanced digestive diseases, such as terminal liver, pancreatic or colon cancer, or chronic pathologies such as decompensated cirrhosis or severe Crohn's disease refractory to treatment.

Palliative care does not aim to cure, but to provide holistic care, taking into account the **physical, psychological, social** and **spiritual** dimensions of suffering. It represents a genuine continuum of care, aimed at preserving patients' dignity and supporting them and their families in the face of the complex challenges posed by an incurable illness. The role of caregivers, particularly nursing assistants, is essential in this context, to **support** the patient in a caring and appropriate way, responding to his or her specific needs in this phase of life.

Relief from physical symptoms

The **physical symptoms** of advanced digestive disease can be extremely distressing. In this context, symptom control is an absolute priority to ensure patient comfort. Palliative care focuses on identifying and treating **uncomfortable** or **painful** symptoms, while taking into account the progression of the disease.

Pain management

Pain is often a major symptom in incurable digestive diseases, particularly digestive cancers (pancreas, liver, stomach). Pain control is therefore a priority. Palliative care uses a range of **analgesics**, from non-steroidal anti-inflammatory drugs to opioids for more intense pain.

Caregivers must be attentive to the **nature of the pain**, its intensity, and the response to treatment. Regular administration of analgesics, with adjustments according to the evolution of pain, is necessary to prevent pain from becoming uncontrollable.

Managing digestive symptoms

In addition to pain, **digestive symptoms** are common and require special attention. Patients with incurable digestive diseases often suffer from :

- **Nausea and vomiting**: These symptoms can be caused by the intestinal obstruction, treatments or the progression of the disease. Palliative care includes the use of antiemetics (anti-nausea drugs) and adapted treatments to relieve these symptoms.
- **Constipation** or **diarrhea**: Caregivers play a crucial role in monitoring and managing transit disorders, which can significantly affect patient comfort.
- **Ascites** (accumulation of fluid in the abdomen): This is common in end-stage liver disease, and can cause significant discomfort. Abdominal drainage (paracentesis) is often necessary to relieve pressure and improve the patient's breathing.
- **Intestinal obstructions**: In some cases, surgery may be contraindicated, and it's essential to manage these symptoms with specific palliative treatments, such as antisecretory drugs or decompression tubes.

Nutrition and hydration

In the advanced stages of the disease, **nutrition** can become a challenge. Patients often lose their appetite or are unable to tolerate a normal diet. Palliative care strives to **reduce the stress associated with eating,** prioritizing comfort over the need to force food intake.

- **Adapted oral nutrition**: Diet should be adapted to the patient's preferences, with frequent light meals or modified textures if necessary.
- **Artificial nutrition**: In some cases, **enteral nutrition** (via nasogastric tube or gastrostomy) or **parenteral nutrition** (intravenous) may be considered. However, it is essential to discuss with the patient and family the appropriateness of continuing this type of nutrition, especially when quality of life becomes a priority.
- **Hydration**: Maintaining adequate hydration is also an important issue, but artificial hydration may be limited in some cases to avoid uncomfortable fluid overload for the patient.

Psychological guidance and emotional support

The **psychological** and **emotional** dimension of palliative care is essential, because faced with an incurable illness, patients are confronted with complex feelings such as **anxiety**, **fear**, **sadness** and even **depression**. Emotional support is an integral part of the palliative approach.

Active listening and empathy

As the closest professional to the patient, the caregiver is often the person who spends the most time with the patient. They need to be attuned to the patient's **worries** and **fears**, while providing constant emotional support.

- **Creating a space to talk**: It's essential that patients can freely express their feelings, fears and questions about the future. Active listening, without judgment or haste, helps patients to feel **understood** and **supported** during this difficult phase.
- **Managing anxiety and depression**: Caregivers can spot signs of emotional distress and, if necessary, seek help from a **psychologist** or **psychiatrist** to provide more

specific support, including appropriate therapies or medication.

Spiritual and social support

In palliative care, **spiritual needs** or reflections on the meaning of life and death often take on increasing importance. For some patients, **spirituality** or **religious convictions** are important resources for coping with the end of life.

- **Spiritual support**: If the patient so wishes, a **spiritual advisor** (priest, chaplain, imam, rabbi, etc.) can be involved in the patient's care. This support can be a way of finding peace and preparing for the end of life with serenity.
- **Maintaining social ties**: It is also essential to support the patient's social ties, by facilitating visits from family and friends. The **social network** is a key factor in improving quality of life at the end of life, and those around them can play a crucial support role, even though they themselves need support.

Family and caregiver support

In palliative care, support involves not only the patient, but also his or her **family** and **caregivers**. They play a crucial role in caring for the patient, but can also be emotionally and physically affected by the burden of care and the anticipation of death.

Helping loved ones accept

Caregivers need to help the family understand the progression of the illness and **accept the reality** of the end of life. This involves open discussion of palliative care goals, including limiting curative treatments and prioritizing comfort.

- **Preparing the family**: It's important to prepare loved ones for what's about to happen, both medically and psychologically. Helping them to anticipate the end-of-life stages can often ease certain anxieties and help them to accept the patient's journey.
- **Early bereavement support**: For families, bereavement often begins before death. Caregivers need to support them through this **period of anticipated grief**, by answering their questions, offering them a space to express their emotions and reassuring them about the care their loved one is receiving.

Home care assistance

If the patient is cared for at home, palliative care includes logistical and technical support for relatives. Caregivers can train the family in certain aspects of **care** (grooming, administering medication), while relieving them of some of the burden.

- **Support for caregivers**: It's important for family caregivers to benefit from **periods of respite**, with the possibility of receiving outside support (care assistants, home nurses, etc.) to avoid exhaustion.

Respecting the patient's dignity and wishes

Respect for the **patient's wishes** and **dignity** is a central component of palliative care. Every patient must be able to express his or her choices concerning the end of life, and these choices must be respected by the care team.

Advance directives and end-of-life choices

In many cases, patients express their **advance wishes** concerning important decisions, such as limiting invasive treatments (mechanical ventilation, resuscitation, etc.) or refusing certain interventions. These directives must be carefully respected, even if they are sometimes difficult for the family or caregivers to accept.

- **Respect for the individual**: Every gesture must be carried out with **respect for** the patient's **dignity**. This includes the way in which care is given, respect for privacy and listening to the patient's preferences, even for simple everyday gestures.

- The caregiver's role in managing pain and comfort at the end of life

The **role of the caregiver in managing pain and comfort at the end of life** is fundamental to ensuring quality care for terminally ill patients. At the end of life, the aim of care is no longer to cure the disease, but to provide **caring support**, relieve pain and provide **physical and emotional comfort**. The caregiver, through his or her daily proximity to the patient, plays an essential role in this process. They act as a link between the patient, his or her loved ones and the nursing team, ensuring that every gesture and every form of care respects the patient's dignity, while alleviating his or her suffering.

Understanding pain at the end of life

Pain is a common symptom in patients at the end of life, particularly those suffering from serious illnesses such as cancer or progressive chronic pathologies. Pain can be **physical**, **psychological** or **emotional**. Understanding the different forms of pain and knowing how to respond to them is crucial to improving the patient's quality of life during this phase.

Types of pain

1. **Physical pain**: This may result from the disease itself (cancer, organ failure) or from the treatments received.

Pain can be acute, chronic or fluctuating, and requires regular assessment to adjust treatments.

2. **Emotional and psychological pain**: Psychological suffering, linked to fear of death, separation anxiety or loss of control, can intensify physical pain. Holistic care must include attention to these non-physical aspects of suffering.

3. **Spiritual pain**: Some patients may express suffering linked to existential or spiritual issues. Although this dimension goes beyond the strictly medical framework, it must be taken into account in the care process.

Pain assessment

The caregiver's primary role in pain management is to be able to **recognize** and **assess** the patient's pain, even when the patient does not express it directly. In many cases, patients, especially at the end of life, may minimize or not verbalize their pain, either out of resignation or fear of adding to the burden of their loved ones.

*   **Use of pain scales**: Caregivers should use **pain assessment scales**, such as the numerical scale (0-10), or behavioral scales for patients unable to communicate verbally, to measure pain intensity. This assessment enables analgesic treatments to be adapted accordingly.
*   **Observing non-verbal signs**: At the end of life, some patients may be too weak to express their pain. Caregivers need to be attentive to **non-verbal signs**, such as grimacing, moaning, agitation or muscle tension. These signals may indicate that the pain is not being properly controlled.

Pain relief: the caregiver's involvement

Pain management is often based on a pharmacological approach, but the caregiver's role goes beyond the simple administration of medication. They are involved in the overall management of the patient's **comfort**, ensuring that treatments are followed, adjusting comfort care and providing psychological support.

Administration of analgesic treatments

Although the administration of drug treatments is often the responsibility of nurses, the nursing auxiliary plays a central role in organizing and monitoring their effectiveness:

- **Treatment monitoring** : Caregivers must ensure that prescribed analgesic treatments (Level 1 to 3 analgesics, opioids, etc.) are administered regularly and as recommended. They must also monitor any side effects, such as opioid-related constipation, and inform the nursing team.
- **Adjusting doses according to pain**: If pain persists despite treatment, the caregiver should inform the nurse or doctor to re-evaluate the care plan. Dose adjustments or the introduction of new drugs may be necessary for better pain control.

Non-pharmacological relief techniques

In addition to medication, caregivers can use **non-pharmacological techniques** to relieve pain and improve patient comfort. These methods can sometimes be just as effective, particularly as a complement to drug treatments.

- **Positioning and mobilization**: Regularly **changing the** patient's **position** can reduce pain associated with immobility or pressure sores. The caregiver must ensure that the patient is positioned comfortably, using support cushions, and that the patient does not remain in the same position for too long.
- **Massages and soothing touch**: A **gentle massage**, without pressure on painful areas, can bring relief and relaxation. **Soothing touch** reassures the patient, creating a bond of closeness and comfort. These simple yet empathetic gestures are often greatly appreciated.
- **Applying heat or cold**: Applying **hot compresses** or **ice packs** can relieve some musculoskeletal or inflammatory pain. These techniques should be used with caution, depending on the patient's condition.

Maintaining overall comfort

Physical comfort is an essential aspect of end-of-life care, and the caregiver plays a key role in adjusting care to improve the patient's quality of life.

- **Hygiene and body care**: The caregiver is responsible for the **cleanliness** and **well-being of** the patient, providing daily hygiene care adapted to the frail state of the patient. Respectful, gentle, non-invasive grooming, and the application of moisturizing creams to prevent irritation, are part of the care that contributes to general comfort.
- **Adapted nutrition and hydration**: At the end of life, a patient's appetite often diminishes. The caregiver can suggest light foods or **nutritional supplements**, respecting the patient's wishes. Hydration must be ensured appropriately, sometimes in the form of small quantities of water or herbal teas, or with mouth care to prevent dry mouth.
- **Pressure sore monitoring**: As the **risk of pressure sores** is high in ridden-bed patients, the caregiver must regularly change the patient's position, use anti-sore mattresses or

cushions, and monitor at-risk areas to prevent pressure sores.

Emotional support and a caring presence

At the end of life, **emotional support** is just as important as physical relief. The caregiver, through his or her daily contact with the patient, often becomes a landmark, a familiar face who offers listening, comfort and **a caring presence**. This role of moral support is crucial in helping the patient to cope with the fears associated with the end of life, and to find a degree of appeasement.

Listening without judging

The caregiver must be attentive to the patient's **concerns** and **emotions**, whether these be fear of death, concern for loved ones, or unexpressed regrets. Being present, without necessarily seeking to provide answers, but offering **active**, empathetic **listening**, is often a source of relief for the patient.

- **Providing a space for expression**: It's important to create a climate of trust in which patients feel free to express their emotions. Caregivers must not minimize concerns, but rather acknowledge them, listen to them and, if necessary, suggest the intervention of a psychologist or spiritual companion.

Promoting a peaceful end to life

The caregiver also helps to organize the moments in life that the patient still wishes to share with loved ones. This may include **preparing for visits**, arranging a more intimate space to encourage exchanges with the family, or simply ensuring that the patient is **comfortably seated** during important moments with loved ones.

Supporting loved ones in managing pain

Pain at the end of life concerns not only the patient, but also their loved ones, who may witness the suffering of their loved one. Caregivers play a crucial role in accompanying families, explaining the care process, reassuring them about pain control, and answering their questions about the end of life.

Informing relatives

Family and friends can sometimes feel **anxious** about their loved one's pain. By explaining palliative care and pain relief measures, the caregiver can help to allay their fears. It's essential to remember that every effort is made to **preserve the** patient's **comfort**.

Supporting families in the final phase

The caregiver's role is also to **support loved ones** as they live out their final moments with the patient. This can include simple gestures such as offering breaks, providing a discreet but reassuring presence, and accompanying them in their own process of acceptance and mourning.

2 Human and psychological support at the end of life

- Listening to and respecting patients' last wishes

Listening to and respecting **patients' last wishes** is a fundamental aspect of end-of-life care. Not only is this an act of respect and dignity, it also helps to alleviate patients' emotional and psychological suffering, while ensuring that they can live out their final moments according to their wishes. At the end of life, patients are often faced with profound questions about their priorities, their values, and how they wish to be cared for. In this delicate phase, careful listening by caregivers and respect for their choices become crucial to ensuring that the end of life is in line with their wishes.

The importance of listening to last wishes

Listening to the patient's last wishes allows us to respect their most intimate wishes regarding the end of their life. Whether it concerns decisions about medical treatment, preferences for place of death, or spiritual or family arrangements, respecting these wishes helps preserve the patient's **dignity** in his or her final moments, and offers a form of control over a process often marked by powerlessness.

Meeting the need for control

At the end of life, many patients express a **need for control** over their situation. This feeling of still being able to decide for themselves, in a context where illness is reducing their autonomy, is often reassuring. Caregivers play a key role in enabling patients to express their wishes, and in ensuring that these are respected as far as possible.

Providing a space for sympathetic listening

Patients at the end of life may have specific requests that go beyond the medical framework: wishes concerning the presence of certain loved ones, religious or spiritual rites, wishes concerning their immediate environment (light, music, silence) or the management of their possessions after their death. For some, it involves decisions about the **medical treatments** they wish to continue or stop, such as stopping invasive procedures, limiting artificial hydration and nutrition, or requesting terminal sedation to relieve pain or anguish.

Respect for medical decisions and advance directives

Patients may have drawn up **advance directives** expressing their wishes in terms of medical treatment, should they no longer be capable of expressing themselves. Advance directives make it possible to anticipate critical situations and ensure that decisions taken by the healthcare team respect the patient's wishes.

Advance directives and trusted third party

Advance directives are an official document in which patients can specify whether or not they wish to undergo certain medical treatments. This can include choices such as refusing to undergo prolonged therapy, stopping resuscitation, or even the wish to receive palliative care to relieve pain without artificially prolonging life. In addition, the patient can designate a **trusted support person** to ensure that these decisions are respected, should the patient become incapable of expressing herself/him.

Informing and advising patients and their families

The role of caregivers is also to **guide** patients and their families through these complex decisions. It's important to clearly explain the implications of each choice, the benefits and limitations of the treatments envisaged, while respecting the patient's priorities. This transparency helps avoid misunderstandings and ensures that the decisions taken correspond to the patient's true wishes.

Respect for personal beliefs and values

The end-of-life stage is a time when personal **values** and **beliefs** become central for patients. Whether religious, philosophical or spiritual, these dimensions must be respected in the care of the patient. Caregivers must show **openness** and constant

benevolence in order to respect the rites, practices or specific needs that stem from these beliefs.

Religious rituals and spiritual practices

Some patients wish to receive specific **religious rites** before their death, such as the presence of a priest for the last rites, or an imam, rabbi or other spiritual companion according to their faith. It is essential to respect these requests and allow the patient to be at peace with his or her beliefs. Similarly, other patients may ask to respect non-religious spiritual practices, such as moments of silence or meditation.

Listening without judging

Caregivers must never **judge** a patient's beliefs, even if they differ from their own. Open-mindedness and non-judgment are essential qualities in providing respectful, soothing care. Patients must feel **free to express** their last wishes without fear of disapproval or misunderstanding.

Taking into account wishes regarding end-of-life location

Where a patient wishes to end his or her life is an important decision. Some patients prefer to **stay in hospital**, where they feel secure in the presence of healthcare professionals. Others wish to return **home**, to be in familiar surroundings surrounded by loved ones, or to specialized units such as palliative care units or hospices.

Home care organization

If a patient expresses the wish to end his or her life at home, caregivers must take the necessary steps to organize **appropriate care at home**. This involves coordinating care at home, ensuring the regular presence of nurses or care assistants, and providing the necessary equipment to maintain the patient's comfort. The caregiver plays a central role in this organization, ensuring that the patient's comfort and dignity are preserved.

Supporting the family in this process

When a patient chooses to die at home, it is essential to support the family too, who may be worried or unsettled by the emotional and practical burden involved. Caregivers can reassure them by training them in simple gestures, offering regular support and reminding them that they can ask for help at any time.

Non-medical last wishes

In addition to medical decisions, patients may have wishes concerning **personal aspects** of their death. These may include details such as the music they wish to hear, the people they wish to see, or more practical arrangements concerning their personal affairs or funeral.

Creating a soothing atmosphere

The caregiver can help to respect these wishes by creating an environment adapted to the patient's wishes. This can include adjusting the lighting, adding soft music, or providing personal objects or photos that comfort the patient. Respecting these small details can make a big difference in helping the patient feel serene in his or her final moments.

Respecting funeral choices

Patients may also express wishes concerning their **funeral** or the management of their body after death (burial, cremation, religious or secular ceremony, donation of the body to science, etc.). Even if these decisions are sometimes beyond the scope of the care team, it is important to collect them and to ensure that loved ones are informed, in order to respect the deceased's last wishes.

- Supporting families at this difficult time

Supporting **families** at the end of a loved one's life is an essential aspect of palliative care. For families, this period is often marked by great emotional suffering, anguish and a sense of powerlessness. They are confronted with the reality of the imminent loss of a loved one, and this stage can be destabilizing, even for those who have prepared for it. Supporting families means more than simply providing medical information: it also means surrounding them with **kindness**, listening to them, and offering them ongoing **emotional support**. The role of caregivers, and in particular nursing assistants, is fundamental in alleviating families' suffering, responding to their needs and enabling them to get through this period more serenely.

The importance of presence and listening

For families, having a caregiver present and listening to them can have a profoundly reassuring effect. They often feel lost or overwhelmed by events, and don't know how to react to their loved one's deteriorating condition. The **simple fact of being there**, offering a sympathetic ear and answering their questions, can reduce their sense of helplessness.

Creating a space for discussion

Families need a **safe space** where they can freely express their worries and fears, as well as their sadness and anger. Caregivers need to create a climate of trust, ensuring that loved ones feel understood and respected in their emotions.

- **Encouraging the expression of feelings**: It's important to remind loved ones that it's normal to feel intense and varied emotions at these difficult times. The caregiver can remind them that there is no "right" way to experience these moments, and that their emotions - whether of sadness, anger or relief - are legitimate.

Reassurance about patient care

One of the main concerns of families is often whether their loved one is suffering, or receiving appropriate care. Caregivers play an essential role in **informing** and **reassuring** loved ones about the quality of the care provided. By explaining the care provided, the treatments administered to relieve pain, and the measures put in place to ensure the patient's comfort, caregivers can help ease families' anxieties.

- **Explain care clearly**: It's essential to provide simple, clear explanations of treatment and care, avoiding medical jargon. This helps relatives to understand what's going on and to feel more involved in the care.
- **Convey a reassuring message**: Even at times when the patient appears unconscious or very weak, it's important to remind loved ones that everything is being done to ensure their loved one's comfort and dignity, and that care is aimed at relieving pain and anxiety.

Helping families make difficult decisions

At the end of life, families are sometimes faced with **difficult decisions**, particularly concerning the continuation or cessation of curative treatments, the use of sedation or measures related to artificial nutrition and hydration. These decisions can be a source of **guilt** and **anguish** for loved ones, who fear making the wrong decisions for their loved one.

Informing medical choices

Caregivers, and in particular the nursing auxiliary, must play a **mediating** role in helping the family to understand what is at stake in these decisions. They must ensure that families have all the information they need to make informed choices, in line with the patient's wishes.

- **Clarifying the objectives of care**: It's crucial that family and friends understand that, in palliative care, the aim is no longer to cure, but to **relieve** and **preserve the** patient's **dignity**. Decisions must be taken within this framework, always respecting the patient's wishes, expressed during his or her lifetime or through advance directives.

- **Supporting without influencing**: The role of caregivers is not to **dictate** decisions to the family, but to provide them with information and support in their reflection. It is essential that family members feel supported in their choices, without outside pressure.

Offer emotional and psychological support

The end of life is often a time of **anticipated bereavement** for loved ones, as they watch their loved one gradually decline. This process can be extremely painful, and families may need psychological support to cope.

Recognizing the pain of loved ones

Caregivers must recognize **families' suffering** and offer them appropriate emotional support. This may mean simply **being present**, listening to their fears and sadness, and offering words of comfort.

- **Easing feelings of guilt**: Families may feel a strong sense of guilt at the idea of not doing enough or not being present enough. The role of the caregiver is to reassure them that they are already doing a great deal for their loved one through their presence and love.
- **Encourage self-care**: In these difficult times, loved ones sometimes tend to forget themselves, neglecting their own well-being in favor of their loved one. It's important to encourage them to take care of themselves, reminding them that they can only support their loved one if they themselves are in good physical and emotional health.

Offer professional psychological help

In some cases, loved ones may need **more specialized psychological support**. The caregiver, in collaboration with the care team, can refer families to a **psychologist** or **spiritual advisor who can** help them get through this period more serenely. These professionals can offer tools for managing anxiety, sadness or anger, and help families prepare for bereavement.

Making farewell moments easier

The last moments of life are often marked by great **emotion**. Families need to be able to **say farewell** to their loved one in a calm, respectful environment, in accordance with the patient's wishes. Caregivers can facilitate these moments by ensuring that families are supported, that the patient is in optimal conditions of comfort, and that exchanges take place in **respectful intimacy**.

Preparing families for the final moments

It's important to support families in the **final stages of** a patient's life. This includes explaining to them the signs of the impending end, anticipating with them what is going to happen, and preparing them for this separation.

- **Inform without rushing**: Caregivers need to find the right words to explain to loved ones what is happening, while respecting their emotional fragility. Families need to know what to expect, but without being overwhelmed by stress or anxiety.

Respecting the privacy of farewells

During the final moments, families often need to **regain intimacy** with their loved one. The caregiver can ensure that these moments take place in a peaceful setting, limiting medical interventions to what is strictly necessary, and offering families the opportunity to spend time with their loved one in an **atmosphere of calm and respect**.

Support after death: mourning support

The role of the caregiver does not end with the patient's death. The **first moments after death** can be particularly difficult for families, and it's important to be there to support them through this transition.

A comforting presence after death

After the death of a loved one, they may be overwhelmed by emotion. The caregiver must support them, offering a **moment's respite**, reassuring them and helping them with the practicalities (calling the funeral home, etc.).

Referral to bereavement support

Bereavement is a long and complex process, and some families will need time to come to terms with the loss of their loved one. The caregiver, in collaboration with the nursing team, can refer families to **support groups or therapists specialized** in bereavement counselling, to offer them a space in which to express their suffering and find support.

Conclusion:

A vocation as a gastroenterology orderly

- Synthesis of necessary skills and day-to-day realities

This **summary of the skills** and **day-to-day realities required** of a nursing assistant highlights the diversity and complexity of this profession, particularly in gastroenterology and palliative care. The nursing auxiliary must combine technical, interpersonal and human skills to provide quality support to patients, while working in close collaboration with the nursing team. This profession, although sometimes misunderstood, is at the heart of patient care, as it lies at the intersection of basic care, comfort and psychological support. Understanding the skills required and the day-to-day realities is essential to grasping the extent of the caregiver's contribution to patient well-being.

Technical skills: ensuring quality basic care

Technical and practical care are at the heart of the caregiver's role. On a day-to-day basis, they provide basic care to ensure patient **comfort**, **cleanliness** and **safety**, while taking care to prevent complications arising from immobility or treatment.

Hygiene and body care management

One of the caregiver's primary responsibilities is to ensure the patient's **hygiene** and **grooming**. These daily tasks are essential to prevent infection, ensure patient comfort and maintain dignity. Whether it's washing in bed, changing clothes or oral hygiene, the caregiver must be gentle, respectful and attentive, so that this care is not perceived as a constraint by the patient.

Preventing complications related to immobility

Bedridden or seriously ill patients, particularly in gastroenterology or palliative care, are often at risk of **complications** such as **bedsores** or respiratory infections. The nursing auxiliary is responsible for :

- **Mobilize the patient regularly** to avoid pressure points and promote blood circulation.
- Use preventive devices such as **anti-bedsore mattresses** or support cushions.
- Make sure the patient is properly positioned, especially after surgery or in the event of abdominal pain, to avoid further discomfort.

Monitoring clinical signs

Although the caregiver is not responsible for medical diagnoses, he or she plays a crucial role in the patient's day-to-day **clinical monitoring**. They must be able to spot signs of deteriorating health, such as abdominal pain, vomiting, fever or signs of dehydration. These observations are then passed on to the nurse or doctor, who will decide what action to take.

Interpersonal skills: an essential human dimension

Interpersonal skills are at the heart of the nursing auxiliary profession. They are often the first point of contact for patients, spending a great deal of time at their bedside. The helping relationship, based on **listening**, **empathy and respect**, is therefore an essential component of the care they provide.

Active listening and communication

Active listening is one of the key interpersonal skills required of a caregiver. Hospitalized patients, especially those with chronic or terminal illnesses, may feel fear, anxiety or loneliness. The caregiver must be able to listen to their concerns, offer them a sympathetic forum, and answer their questions in a reassuring manner.

Communication is not limited to exchanges with patients, but also extends to collaboration with **care teams**. The caregiver is often the one who passes on essential information about the patient's progress, which can influence medical decisions. Good communication with doctors, nurses and other caregivers is therefore essential to ensure smooth, consistent care.

Psychological support and empathy

Caregivers also play a crucial role in providing **emotional support** to patients, especially those at times of great vulnerability, such as palliative care patients or those suffering from incurable digestive diseases. **Empathy** is an indispensable quality for understanding patients' emotional needs and helping them feel heard and supported. At the end of life, this comforting presence enables patients to find a degree of relief, even when words fail them.

Organizational skills: efficiency and adaptation

The daily routine of a nursing auxiliary is marked by an **intense rhythm**. They juggle a large number of patients, a variety of care tasks, and often unforeseen situations. This means they need to **be** highly **organized** and **adaptable** to ensure quality care, often within a limited timeframe.

Managing priorities

Every day, the caregiver has to assess and **prioritize**. Patients in critical situations require more urgent attention, but comfort care for other patients must not be neglected. Managing priorities requires the ability to quickly assess situations and make appropriate decisions.

Adapting to the unexpected

In the hospital environment, the unexpected is a frequent occurrence. Whether it's a sudden complication, a change in treatment or a medical emergency, caregivers need to know how to **manage stress** and **adapt** quickly to new situations. This responsiveness is essential to meet patients' changing needs.

Day-to-day realities: a job of dedication and endurance

Being a caregiver means facing realities that are often physically and psychologically demanding. The days are long, the work is sometimes arduous, and contact with suffering, illness and death can be hard to bear. Despite this, it's a profession that also brings a great deal of **satisfaction** and **meaning**, because it's based on the values of **caring for others**, **dedication** and **human solidarity**.

Physical and emotional fatigue

Caregivers are often confronted with **physical fatigue**, due in particular to staggered working hours and repetitive tasks such as patient mobilization or body care. Managing these efforts requires good physical condition and **techniques to prevent musculoskeletal disorders**, such as adopting the right postures during care.

Emotional fatigue is also a daily reality, particularly in departments where patient suffering is omnipresent, such as palliative care. Watching patients suffer or die can be psychologically taxing, and caregivers must learn to strike a balance between **emotional closeness** and **professional distance** to preserve their own mental health.

The importance of recognition and teamwork

Despite these challenges, caregivers derive great satisfaction from their work, largely due to the positive impact they can have on **patients' quality of life**. Being recognized and appreciated by patients and their families is a source of **motivation** and **pride**.

Teamwork is also one of the enriching realities of daily life. Collaboration with nurses, doctors and other healthcare professionals creates a **mutually supportive environment**, where each can rely on the other to provide the best possible care.

- Encouragement to persevere and get involved in this specialty

Choosing to become a nursing auxiliary, particularly in gastroenterology or in demanding departments such as palliative care, is a choice that requires **courage**, **determination** and a deep vocation for caring for others. It's a path that's often perceived as trying, and sometimes misunderstood in all its magnitude, but in return it offers immeasurable **human riches**. While this specialty may seem difficult, even intimidating at first glance, it is also a source of **pride** and **satisfaction** for those who choose it and dedicate themselves to it. Persevering in this specialty, despite the challenges, is an approach that deserves to be encouraged, as it opens the door to a career in which every gesture has a **direct and precious impact** on patients' lives.

The importance of an essential contribution

Every member of the healthcare team plays a crucial role, but the caregiver is often the one closest to the patient. He or she provides a fundamental link between the patient and the rest of the medical team, as the one who observes, takes care of the most immediate needs and is able to offer **ongoing support**. In gastroenterology, for example, where pathologies can be disabling and burdensome, the caregiver is a presence of **comfort** and **stability**, and sometimes the last line of defence against physical and psychological pain.

Involvement in this specialty means accepting to play a decisive role in the patient's **daily well-being**. Even if certain tasks may seem repetitive, such as grooming or changing position, they are fundamental to preserving the **dignity** and **comfort** of those being cared for. Patients, often faced with complex illnesses or demanding treatments, depend on the vigilance and attentive care of the caregiver to maintain a certain quality of life. In palliative care, where support towards the end of life is a central concern, the caregiver enables patients to live out their final moments in **dignity** and **serenity**, far from unnecessary suffering.

Overcoming challenges to grow

There's no denying that this specialty presents challenges, whether physical, emotional or organizational. Fatigue linked to staggered working hours, managing patients in critical situations, or constant exposure to suffering are realities that every caregiver has to face. Yet these challenges are also **opportunities for growth**.

- **Growing in the face of responsibility**: Every difficult situation helps to develop essential skills, whether stress management, rapid decision-making or adaptability in unforeseen situations. Through these experiences, caregivers hone their ability to work under pressure while remaining attentive to patients' needs. This responsibility, though sometimes overwhelming, is a source of great **professional pride**.

- **Gaining in humanity**: Working in contact with vulnerable patients and families facing illness or the end of life enables **us** to develop **deep empathy** and **understanding of others**. Proximity to the deepest human realities - suffering, fear, death - gives a unique perspective on life and on the meaning of the profession. The caregiver learns to listen beyond words, to offer a reassuring presence even in the darkest moments, and to understand that, sometimes, simply being there is the greatest comfort.

Impact on the lives of others: a powerful motivator

Every day, the caregiver has the opportunity to **positively influence** patients' lives, whether by relieving pain, providing

393

comfort, or simply offering a smile and an attentive ear. This direct impact on patients' well-being is a source of **daily motivation**. Every gesture, no matter how small, can make a difference to a patient who is feeling vulnerable or alone.

The thanks of patients and their families, often touched by the caregiver's humanity and benevolence, are concrete testimony to the importance of this work. It is often said that patients remember the little touches and gestures of care more than the technical medical acts. This power to improve quality of life, even in difficult circumstances, is a **powerful driving force** for continuing and persevering in this way.

Training and enrichment in a constantly evolving specialty

Gastroenterology and palliative care are **constantly evolving** fields, where new technologies, medical advances and new approaches to care are regularly changing practices. Involvement in this specialty also means choosing to continue **learning**, training and enriching oneself throughout one's career. Each new skill acquired strengthens the caregiver's ability to offer appropriate care, understand new techniques, and stay as close as possible to patients' needs.

Specific training courses, whether in pain management, digestive care techniques or end-of-life care, enable the development of invaluable **know-how** that makes the nursing auxiliary a key player in the care team. By constantly upgrading their skills, caregivers enrich their expertise and become an indispensable element in the continuous improvement of care.

A meaningful profession: choosing to support people

One of the main reasons why it's essential to persevere and get involved in this specialty is that it's a profession that gives **deep meaning** to one's professional life. Devoting one's time and energy to **caring for others**, alleviating their suffering and accompanying them in moments of great vulnerability, is meaningful work that brings not only professional satisfaction, but also **personal richness**.

Unlike other professions, where the impact of one's work may seem abstract or remote, the caregiver sees the concrete results of his or her commitment every day. This **human dimension** of the profession is irreplaceable. By choosing to invest oneself fully in this specialty, we choose to have a direct and positive impact on the lives of others, which is both gratifying and inspiring.

- The importance of caring and respect for the patient

Caring and **respect** for the patient are two fundamental principles of the care-giver-patient relationship, particularly in the healthcare sector. These values are not limited to simple attitudes or forms of politeness: they are at the very heart of the quality of care provided, influencing both the physical and psychological well-being of the patient, as well as the overall effectiveness of the care provided. For a caregiver, in particular, kindness and respect are essential pillars of daily work, as they help build a relationship of trust with the patient, humanize care, and contribute to the patient's **dignity** in moments of vulnerability. To engage in this approach is not only to meet patients' medical needs, but also to **honor their humanity**.

Benevolence: continuous attention to patient well-being

Benevolence in care isn't just a matter of courtesy, it's a global attitude that puts the patient at the center of everything we do, anticipating his or her needs and ensuring his or her comfort. As a caregiver, this benevolence translates into a multitude of small attentions which, taken together, considerably improve the patient's quality of life.

Gentle, patient care

In a context where suffering, pain and anxiety are often omnipresent, it is essential that every gesture is marked by **gentleness** and **patience**. Patients, especially those with chronic illnesses or in palliative care, can be both physically and psychologically **fragile**. Every act of care, whether it's bathing, changing position or simply taking a blood pressure, must be carried out with the kindness that reassures and soothes.

- **Adapting to the patient's rhythm**: It's important to adapt to the patient's rhythm, avoiding rushing or executing actions mechanically. For example, when the patient is in pain, the caregiver must adjust his or her actions to limit discomfort, taking care to communicate with the patient at every stage of care.
- **Anticipating needs**: Being caring also means knowing how to **anticipate** a patient's needs, sometimes even before he or she expresses them. This may involve simple gestures such as adjusting a pillow, checking the room temperature, or offering water without the patient having to ask for it.

Offering a comforting presence

Benevolence also implies a **reassuring presence**, an emotional availability that allows the patient to feel supported, even in the most difficult moments. This presence doesn't necessarily require big words or spectacular actions; sometimes, simply being there, listening, and showing empathy is enough to make the patient feel that he's not alone in his struggle.

- **Active listening**: Patients often need to express their fears, pain or questions. Listening attentively, without interruption or judgment, is a sign of kindness that helps reduce feelings of isolation.
- **Providing moral support**: Patients, especially when faced with a serious illness, can feel helpless in the face of

uncertainty. By showing **understanding** and **support**, the caregiver can help them find comfort. Simply saying "I'm here for you" can sometimes be enough to lighten the patient's load.

Respect: preserving the patient's dignity

Respect for the patient is demonstrated through all interactions, gestures and care provided. Respecting patients means recognizing and **honoring their dignity**, even at times when they may feel diminished by illness or old age. This respect is essential to maintaining a relationship of trust and ensuring that the patient feels valued and taken into account.

Respecting privacy and autonomy

Care, whether technical or relational, must always **respect the** patient's **privacy**. Even when we are called upon to intervene in very personal aspects of the patient's life, such as toileting, changing clothes or monitoring catheters, it is vital to protect his or her privacy. This involves simple gestures such as closing the bedroom door, using screens, or covering certain parts of the body during care.

- **Explaining every gesture**: Another aspect of respect is clearly **explaining** every gesture or treatment to the patient, so that he or she understands what's going on and doesn't feel dispossessed of his or her own body. Respecting patients' autonomy also means asking for their agreement before any action is taken, even for routine gestures.
- **Respecting patient choice**: Whenever possible, it is essential to let the patient **decide** what care he or she wishes to receive. For example, a patient at the end of life may choose to limit invasive treatments or refuse certain care. Respecting these choices, even if they run counter to the traditional approach to care, is a sign of respect for the patient's wishes and dignity.

Valuing the individual beyond the disease

It's easy, especially in a hospital or long-term care setting, to see patients solely in terms of their illness or condition. Yet respecting patients also means seeing them as **unique individuals**, with their own stories, emotions and values. Illness does not define the whole patient, and it's important to always remember that behind every diagnosis lies a person who deserves **consideration** and **appreciation**.

- **Personalizing care**: Every patient is different, and it's crucial not to fall into a one-size-fits-all approach to care. Personalizing care, taking into account individual preferences, habits and needs, is a form of respect. For example, making sure that meals correspond to the patient's tastes or restrictions, or adapting care to the patient's lifestyle.
- **Respecting beliefs and values**: Respect also means recognizing patients' **beliefs**, **values** and **preferences**, whether religious, cultural or personal. This means not imposing a single vision of care, but integrating the patient's wishes into the treatment process.

The benefits of caring and respect for patients and caregivers

Benevolence and respect for the patient are not only beneficial for the patient; they also have a positive impact on the entire care team and on the overall quality of care.

Improving patient well-being

When patients feel respected and cared for, they feel more comfortable expressing their needs, pains and concerns. This climate of **mutual trust** fosters better communication between caregiver and patient, which can lead to more effective and appropriate care.

- **Reduced stress and anxiety**: A patient who feels cared for, listened to and understood is often less anxious, which improves his or her general well-being. Knowing that one's needs will be taken into account and one's wishes respected helps patients feel more secure, even in difficult situations.

Personal enrichment for the caregiver

Caring and respect are **enriching values** for the caregiver. By adopting a human-centered approach, caregivers develop valuable **emotional** and **relational skills** that go beyond the technical. This gives greater **meaning** to daily work, and provides real professional satisfaction in the knowledge that every gesture has a positive impact.

A calm working climate

Respect and benevolence also contribute to a **calm climate** within care teams. When these values are shared and applied by all staff, relations between colleagues and with patients improve. This fosters greater **team cohesion**, reduces tension and improves quality of life at work.

Appendices

- Glossary of medical terms in gastroenterology

Here's a **glossary of medical terms in gastroenterology**, covering key concepts, pathologies, procedures and symptoms frequently encountered in this specialty.

A

- **Abdomen**: Part of the body between the thorax and pelvis, containing many organs of the digestive system (stomach, intestines, liver, etc.).
- **Adhesions**: Bands of scar tissue that form between abdominal organs, often following surgery or inflammation, which can cause pain or obstruction.
- **Anastomosis**: Surgical connection between two hollow organ segments, often used after resection of part of the intestine.
- **Anorexia**: Loss or reduction of appetite, often associated with digestive pathologies or heavy treatments (such as chemotherapy).
- **Ascites**: accumulation of fluid in the abdominal cavity, often caused by cirrhosis or heart failure.

B

- **Bloating**: Sensation of abdominal swelling, often due to the accumulation of gas in the intestines.
- Biopsy: Removal of a tissue sample for microscopic examination, often used to diagnose diseases such as cancer or inflammatory diseases.
- **Bilirubin**: Yellow pigment resulting from the breakdown of hemoglobin, excreted by the liver. An increase in bilirubin in the blood can cause jaundice.
- **Boerhaave syndrome**: Spontaneous rupture of the esophagus, often caused by violent vomiting.

C

- **Cirrhosis**: Chronic liver disease characterized by excessive fibrosis (scarring) of liver tissue, leading to progressive loss of liver function.
- **Cholangitis**: Inflammation of the bile ducts, often due to obstruction caused by stones or infection.
- **Cholecystectomy**: Surgical removal of the gallbladder, usually for symptomatic gallstones.
- **Colitis**: Inflammation of the colon, often present in diseases such as ulcerative colitis.
- **Colonoscopy**: Visual examination of the inner lining of the colon using an endoscope, to diagnose diseases such as polyps, diverticula or colon cancer.
- **Crohn's disease**: chronic inflammatory bowel disease that can affect any part of the digestive tract, causing abdominal pain, diarrhea and weight loss.

D

- **Diverticulum**: Small pouch that forms in the wall of the intestine, often in the colon. Inflammation of a diverticulum is called diverticulitis.
- **Dyspepsia**: General term to describe a set of digestive symptoms such as abdominal pain, nausea and bloating, often after meals.
- **Dysphagia**: difficulty swallowing, a frequent symptom of esophageal pathologies.

E

- **Endoscopy**: Technique for visually examining the inside of hollow organs (such as the stomach or esophagus) using a flexible tube fitted with a camera.
- **Enteritis**: Inflammation of the small intestine, often caused by infection, autoimmune disease or radiation.
- **Eructation**: Expulsion of gas through the mouth, commonly called "burping".
- **Evisceration**: Protrusion of internal organs through an opening in the abdominal wall, usually following injury or surgery.

F

- **Hepatic fibrosis**: Accumulation of scar tissue in the liver following repeated damage, which can progress to cirrhosis.
- **Fistula**: Abnormal passage between two hollow organs or between an organ and the body surface, often as a result of infection or surgery.

G

- **Gastrectomy**: Partial or total removal of the stomach, usually for gastric cancer.
- **Gastroenteritis**: Inflammation of the stomach and intestines, often due to a viral or bacterial infection, causing diarrhea, vomiting and abdominal pain.
- **Gastroscopy**: visual examination of the stomach using an endoscope, often performed to diagnose ulcers, gastritis or gastric cancer.
- **Glutenopathy**: Intolerance to gluten, also known as celiac disease, leading to inflammation of the small intestine in people sensitive to gluten.

H

- **Hematemesis**: Vomiting blood, often due to upper digestive hemorrhage (esophagus, stomach, duodenum).
- Hemorrhoids: Dilated veins in the rectum or anus, often responsible for pain and bleeding.
- **Hepatitis**: Inflammation of the liver, which may be viral, alcoholic or autoimmune in origin.
- **Hernia**: Protrusion of an organ or part of an organ through a muscular or tissue wall, often in the abdomen.

I

- **Icterus**: Yellow discoloration of the skin and mucous membranes due to an accumulation of bilirubin in the blood, often linked to liver or biliary tract disease.

- **Ileus**: Stopped intestinal peristalsis, often associated with intestinal obstruction or bowel paralysis after abdominal surgery.
- **Inflammation**: The body's immune response to aggression, characterized by redness, heat, swelling and pain, often seen in inflammatory bowel disease.

L

- **Biliary lithiasis**: Presence of stones in the gallbladder or bile ducts, often responsible for biliary colic or cholecystitis.
- **Liver function tests**: A set of blood tests used to assess liver function, such as liver enzyme levels (ALAT, ASAT) or bilirubin.

M

- **Melena**: Black, tarry stools, a sign of upper digestive hemorrhage.
- **Metaplasia**: Transformation of one type of tissue into another type of abnormal tissue, often observed in precancerous lesions such as Barrett's esophagus.

N

- **Nausea**: Sensation of discomfort or the need to vomit, common in digestive diseases.
- **Necrosis**: Death of cells or tissues, often due to lack of blood supply or infection.

O

- **Intestinal obstruction**: Obstruction of the intestine preventing the normal passage of digestive contents, caused by adhesions, tumors or hernias.
- **Esophagitis**: Inflammation of the lining of the esophagus, often caused by gastroesophageal reflux disease.

P

- **Pancreatitis**: Inflammation of the pancreas, which can be acute or chronic, often linked to gallstones or alcoholism.
- **Digestive perforation**: Rupture of a hollow organ in the digestive tract, requiring urgent surgical intervention.
- **Polyp**: An abnormal mass of tissue that develops on the inner wall of an organ, such as the colon, often benign but sometimes precancerous.
- **Proctology**: Branch of medicine specializing in the diagnosis and treatment of diseases of the anus and rectum.

R

- **Gastroesophageal reflux disease (GERD)**: backflow of acidic gastric fluid into the esophagus, causing burning and retrosternal pain.
- **Resection**: Surgical removal of part of an organ, often for cancer or inflammatory diseases.

S

- **Hepatic sclerosis**: Another term for cirrhosis, an advanced stage of liver fibrosis.
- **Sigmoiditis**: Inflammation of the sigmoid portion of the colon, often associated with diverticula.
- **Stenosis**: Narrowing of a duct or organ, as in the case of intestinal stenosis due to Crohn's disease.

T

- **Liver transplantation**: Replacement of the diseased liver with a healthy donor liver, the ultimate treatment for end-stage liver disease.
- **Tumor**: An abnormal mass of cells, which may be benign or malignant, frequently observed in digestive cancers.

U

- **Ulcerative colitis (ulcerative colitis)**: Chronic inflammatory disease of the colon characterized by ulcers on the colonic mucosa, causing bloody diarrhea and abdominal pain.

V

- **Esophageal varices**: Dilatations of the veins of the esophagus, often caused by portal hypertension, which can lead to serious bleeding.
- **Volvulus**: Torsion of part of the intestine, causing acute intestinal obstruction requiring surgery.

Z

- **Zollinger-Ellison syndrome**: Rare disease characterized by excessive gastrin secretion, leading to refractory gastric ulcers.

This glossary covers the main terms used in **gastroenterology**, providing a solid foundation for understanding the diseases, treatments and symptoms in this specialty.

- Practical sheets for ostomy management, enteral nutrition

Here are some **practical information sheets** on **ostomy care** and **enteral nutrition**. These sheets are designed to provide concrete, detailed information for caregivers, enabling them to fully understand and master these specific aspects of care.

1. Practical guide: Ostomy management

Definition of an ostomy

A **stoma** is a surgical opening created to divert intestinal or urinary contents outside the body. Stomas can be temporary or permanent, depending on the underlying pathology. The main stomas include :

- **Colostomy**: Opening of the colon through the skin to divert stool.

- Ileostomy: Cutting of the ileum (small intestine) through the skin to divert stool.
- **Urostomy**: Abduction of the urinary tract through the skin to divert urine.

Management objectives

- Ensure good stoma hygiene.
- Prevent complications (infections, skin irritations).
- Ensuring patient comfort and dignity.
- Ensure patient autonomy in stoma management, if possible.

Materials required

- Ostomy pouch adapted to the type of stoma (colostomy, ileostomy, urostomy).
- Skin protectors and sealing rings.
- Sterile compresses.
- Warm water and mild soap to clean the skin around the stoma.
- Non-sterile gloves.
- Scissors to adjust pocket cut-out.
- Adhesive tape for fixing if necessary.

Stages of care

1. **Material preparation**: Have all the necessary instruments ready before you start. Make sure the patient is comfortable and informed about the treatment steps.

2. **Removing the old pocket** :
   - Gently remove the pouch, holding the skin with one hand to avoid pulling on the stoma.
   - Inspect the skin around the stoma for redness, irritation or signs of infection.
   - Clean the area with lukewarm water and mild soap. Avoid aggressive products.

3. **Ostomy cleaning** :

   ○ Use a water-soaked compress to gently clean around the stoma. Gently pat dry with a clean compress.
   ○ Check the color of the stoma. A healthy stoma should be pink or red, with no excessive bleeding.

4. **Preparing the new pouch** :

   ○ Cut the new pouch to fit the size and shape of the stoma. Make sure the opening is just big enough to surround the stoma without leaving too much skin exposed.
   ○ Apply a skin protector around the stoma to avoid irritation.

5. **Laying the new pocket** :

   ○ Apply the new pouch, pressing firmly around the stoma to ensure a good seal.
   ○ Check that the bag is secure and comfortable for the patient.

6. **Patient education** :

   ○ If possible, teach the patient how to change the ostomy pouch and how to monitor for complications.
   ○ Explain the importance of good hygiene and skin monitoring.

Complications to watch out for

- **Skin irritations**: Signs of redness, itching or pain around the stoma. Prevent by using skin protectors.
- **Parastomal hernia**: Swelling around the stoma, requiring medical assessment.
- **Stoma necrosis**: Appearance of a black or purplish color, a sign of poor vascularization.
- **Pocket leakage**: Signs of poor pocket fit or incorrect cutting, requiring revision of size or fitting technique.

2. Practical info: enteral nutrition

Definition of enteral nutrition

Enteral nutrition involves administering nutrients directly into the digestive tract via a tube (nasogastric, gastrostomy or jejunostomy) when the patient is unable to eat orally but the digestive tract is still functioning.

Management objectives

- Ensure adequate nutritional intake to maintain health and avoid malnutrition.
- Ensure safe and hygienic handling of probes and nutrients.
- Prevent complications associated with enteral nutrition (tube occlusion, infection, regurgitation).

Materials required

- Nasogastric tube, gastrostomy or jejunostomy.
- Enteral nutrition pump or syringe for gravity feeding.
- Sachets or pouches of nutrient solution.
- Sterile water for rinsing.
- Compresses and fastening material.
- Non-sterile gloves.

Stages of care

1. **Material preparation :**

   - Wash your hands and wear gloves.
   - Prepare the prescribed nutrient solution (check expiry date and ambient temperature).
   - Install the equipment (pump or syringe) and ensure that the probe is correctly positioned and secured.

2. **Checking the probe** :

   ◦ Make sure the probe is in place and working properly. If the probe is nasogastric, check its position by suction or X-ray before each use.
   ◦ For a gastrostomy or jejunostomy, check the skin around the tube for signs of infection or irritation.

3. **Administration of nutrition** :

   ◦ **Gravity** feed: Use a syringe to slowly feed the solution into the probe.
   ◦ **Pump** administration: Connect the nutrition bag to the pump, set the flow rate and ensure that the solution flows at the prescribed rate.
   ◦ Duration and flow rate must be respected to avoid digestive complications (vomiting, bloating).

4. **Rinsing the probe** :

   ◦ Rinse the probe with sterile water before and after each administration to avoid obstructions.
   ◦ Use a syringe containing 20-30 ml sterile water to clean the probe.

5. **Monitoring during feeding** :

   ◦ Monitor the patient's condition during and after administration (nausea, abdominal pain, regurgitation, etc.).
   ◦ Regularly check food tolerance (absence of bloating, diarrhea or constipation).
   ◦ Watch for signs of dehydration and ensure adequate water intake.

Complications to watch out for

- **Probe obstruction**: Occurs if the probe is not properly rinsed after each use. If obstruction is suspected, try rinsing with lukewarm or sterile water.
- **Regurgitation and false route**: Watch for signs of coughing, choking or cyanosis during administration. In

the event of a false route, stop feeding immediately and alert the medical team.

- **Tube site infection**: In case of gastrostomy or jejunostomy, monitor the area around the tube for signs of infection (redness, warmth, discharge).

Tips for caregivers

- **Patient and family education**: If the patient is at home, make sure the family understands how to administer nutrition, clean the tube, and recognize complications.
- **Strict hygiene**: Always ensure rigorous hygiene when handling the probe and nutrient solutions to avoid infection.

Managing **ostomies** and **enteral nutrition** requires constant vigilance, good technique and the ability to anticipate and manage complications. Caregivers' involvement in patient education is also crucial to guaranteeing autonomy and comfort in these situations.

- References and resources for caregivers

Here is a selection of **useful reading references** and **resources** for caregivers, covering various aspects of the profession, from basic care to specific skills, palliative care support and patient communication. These resources can be used to deepen knowledge, improve practices and better understand certain clinical situations.

Books for caregivers

1. **"A practical guide for caregivers**
   Author : *Corinne Foucher*
   Description : This guide is a reference for caregivers. It covers all practical aspects of the profession, from basic care to patient communication and emergency

management. It is designed to be accessible, with clear explanations and plenty of advice for everyday practice.

2. **"Basic hospital care**
Author : *Laurence Leautier*
Description : This book offers a complete presentation of basic care in the hospital environment, aimed at care assistants. It details essential technical gestures, such as toileting, hygiene care, position changes and emergency care, while touching on human aspects such as listening and communication.

3. **"The caregiver-caregiver relationship: Issues, perspectives and practices"**
Author : *Brigitte Sandrin-Berthon*
Description : This book emphasizes the importance of the human relationship between caregiver and patient. It explores the different dimensions of this relationship (communication, empathy, emotional management) and provides practical tools for improving the quality of care.

4. **"Palliative care manual for caregivers"**
Author: *Elisabeth Kübler-Ross*
Description : An indispensable manual for palliative care assistants, with explanations on accompanying patients at the end of life, pain management, psychological support and caring for families. It emphasizes the importance of caring and respect during this delicate period.

5. **"Home care techniques for caregivers"**
Author : *Christian Leroy*
Description : This book is specifically designed for homecare assistants. It offers methods and advice for organizing home care, managing chronic or dependent patients, and assisting families with day-to-day management.

Articles and trade magazines

1. **"Soins aides-soignantes" (Monthly magazine)**
   Description: This magazine is aimed specifically at caregivers, and each month features articles on changes in practices, the latest recommendations, case studies and feedback from caregivers in the field.

2. **"La revue francophone de gériatrie et gérontologie" (The French-speaking journal of geriatrics and gerontology)**
   Description : An excellent resource for caregivers working with the elderly. The magazine covers topics such as caring for people at the end of life, preventing falls, specific care for age-related pathologies, and pressure sore management.

3. **"Le Journal des Soins Infirmiers**
   Description : Although this journal is primarily aimed at nurses, it is also an excellent resource for nursing aides, particularly when it comes to care protocols, technological innovations and patient safety recommendations.

Websites and online resources

1. **ANFH (Association Nationale pour la Formation permanente du personnel Hospitalier)**
   Website
   Description: This site offers a wide range of **continuing training courses** for nursing assistants, particularly in specific areas such as geriatric patient management, palliative care and the prevention of nosocomial infections.

2. **Nurses.com**
   Website
   Description: This site offers a wide range of resources for caregivers, including articles on clinical practice, videos

explaining technical procedures, discussion forums for exchanging experiences, and information on the latest innovations in the field of care.

3. **HAS (Haute Autorité de Santé)**
    Website
    Description: The HAS provides guides and recommendations for healthcare professionals, including care assistants. These include care protocols, recommendations on chronic patient management and information on good palliative care practices.

4. **Aide-soignant guide (Fédération Hospitalière de France)**
    Website
    Description: The Fédération Hospitalière de France website offers a **guide dedicated to orderlies**, with practical information on the orderly's job, technical fact sheets and advice on how to fit into a hospital team.

5. **Fondation de France - Palliative care fund**
    Website
    Description : The Fondation de France offers resources to support caregivers in palliative care, with practical guides and educational documents on accompanying patients at the end of life.

Training and certification

1. **Espace Compétences (South of France) - Caregiver training**
    Website
    Description : Offers **ongoing training** for nursing assistants, with modules on topics such as caring for patients with chronic illnesses, pain management and managing stress in the workplace.

2. **Pôle emploi - Training for caregivers**
   Website
   Description: The Pôle emploi website lists specialized training courses for care assistants, particularly in home care, support for the elderly or dying, and new care techniques.

Useful mobile applications

1. **iStoma**
   Description: Application dedicated to caregivers of ostomy patients. It features technical data sheets, videos explaining ostomy placement and care, and practical advice to improve patients' quality of life.

2. **Nutrition+**
   Description: This application offers resources on **clinical** and **enteral nutrition**, with automatic calculations of nutritional requirements and guides for adapting patients' diets to their state of health.

3. **e-Hospices**
   Description: Mobile application offering advice and recommendations for managing palliative **care** patients, plus access to articles, videos and feedback from experts in the field.

These resources will help you deepen your skills, keep up to date with the latest care practices and support you in your work as a caregiver. **Ongoing training**, access to specialized reading and sharing your experience with other professionals will enable you to perfect your skills and offer patients the most appropriate and respectful care.